Daoist Qigong

The Art of "Inner" Alchemy

by Igor Dudukchan

The Qigong it is a Chinese art of management of the internal energy Qi. Qigong has much different schools and directions.

The outlined Qigong method in this book was originated in Tianzhu Shan mountains and was developed by such famous Daoist masters as Ling Gu, He Jiafan, Wang Jiafan, Liang Yaopin. Its modern form, this system got due to the efforts of such mentor as Liu Shaobin.

A distinctive feature of the presented to the readers system is the harmonious combination of static and dynamic exercises, which allows easily and relatively quickly achieve tangible results in the mastering of the ancient Daoist art of the "Inner alchemy".

© 2017, Dudukchan I.M.
All Rights reserved.
Author: Igor Dudukchan
Translator: Marina Kondratenko
ISBN: 9781520710662

Contents:

Introduction

The traditional Chinese medicine and the **Qigong** (the art of the control of the energy Qi) pay a little attention to the anatomy in the modern Western understanding and make the accent on the functions of the physical organs. The ancient mendicants and the masters of Qigong thought that it is important to own the specific Qi energy for the normal functioning of the organs. According to the traditional Chinese beliefs, there is the energy of two types in the organism: inner and outer, and each of the types of the energy cycles along their own ways. The outer Qi comes through the breathing from outside into the organism of the person. The inner Qi is the energy which cycles inside the person's body.

During the breathing the outer Qi gets into the organism of the person, partly becoming the inner Qi and goes outside at the exit and becomes the outer Qi again.

This way the constant circulation of the Qi energy is made through the certain meridians (**Jinglo**).

In the theory of the Chinese medicine and the Qigong the 12 main paired meridians are underlined (Fig. 1-12), 8 "wonderful" meridians (the most important: the frontal-medium meridian (The Conception Vessel Meridian) of the action - **Ren-mai** (fig. 13) and the backward-medium meridian (The Governing Vessel Meridian) of the control - Du-mai (fig. 14) and 15 secondary meridians. There are the specific points on the way of the movement of each meridian. The pressure on these points influences on the functioning of the whole meridian. These points are called the acupuncture points.

Let's list the main acupuncture points.

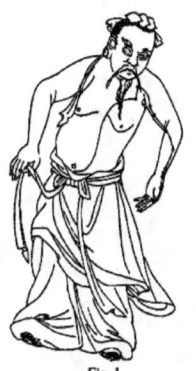

Fig.1
The Lung meridian

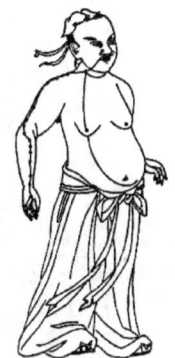

Fig.2
The Large Intestine meridian

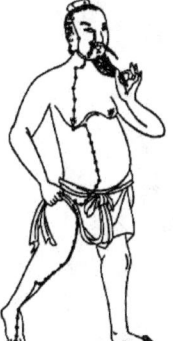

Fig.3
The stomach meridian

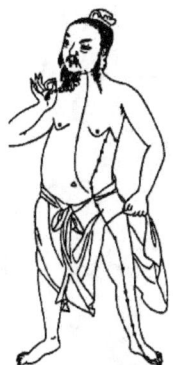

Fig.4
The Spleen meridian

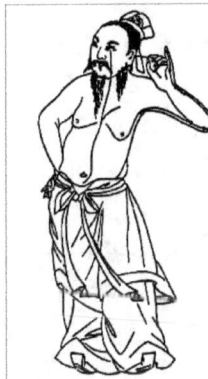

Fig.5
The Heart meridian

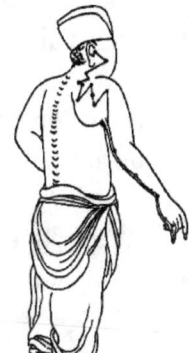

Fig.6
The Small Intestine meridian

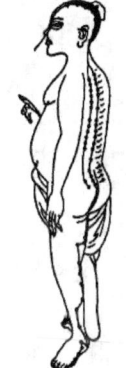

Fig.7
The Urinary bladder meridian

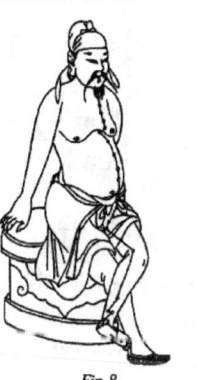

Fig.8
The Kidney meridian

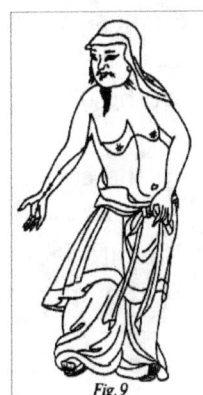

Fig.9
The Pericardium meridian

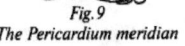

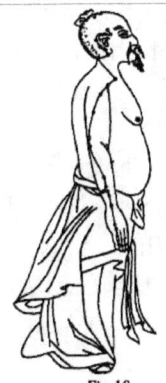

Fig.10
The Sanjiao meridian

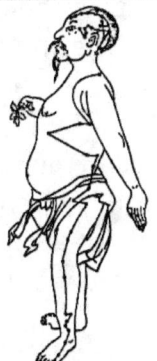

Fig.11
The Gall bladder meridian

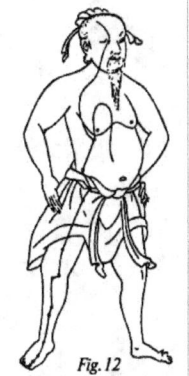

Fig.12
The Liver meridian

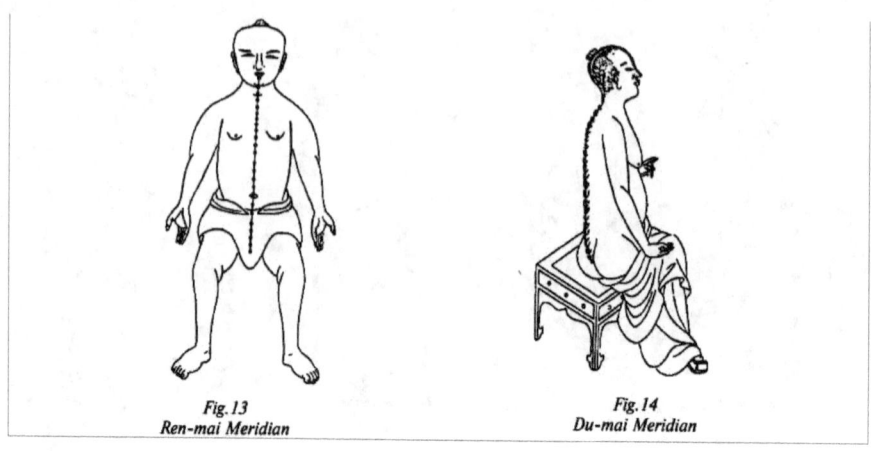

Fig. 13
Ren-mai Meridian

Fig. 14
Du-mai Meridian

The acupuncture points on the frontal part of the head
(fig. 15):

Shenting – GV24 (The yard of the spirit) is located on the midline of the head, 1,2 cm upper the frontal border of the growth of the hair.

Tianmu (The sky eye) is located on the midline of the forehead, above the Yintang at a distance equal to the width of the eye socket from its medial to the lateral border.

Yintang (The print hall) is located midway between the eyebrows. In the center of the nose bridge. In the middle of the line connecting the inner ends of the eyebrows.

Suliao – GV25 (The just hole) is located on the tip of the nose.
Renzhong - Du26 (The middle of the man) is located under the nasal septum in the upper third of the vertical grooves of the upper lip.

Cheng jiang – CV24 (The juice collecting) is located in the cavity below the lower lip, in the center of chin-labial furrows.

Yinjiao (The center of the gum) (fig. 16) is located at the interface of the mucosa of the upper lip to the gum (frenulum of the upper lip).

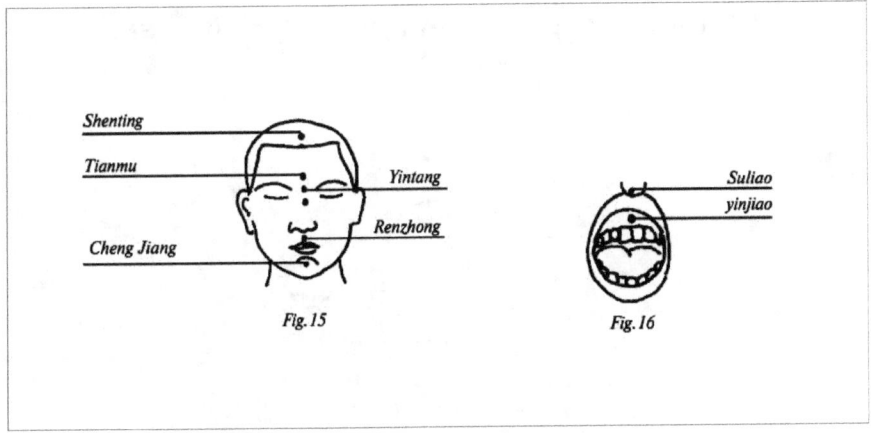

Fig. 15   Fig. 16

Acupuncture points on the top of the head
(fig. 17):

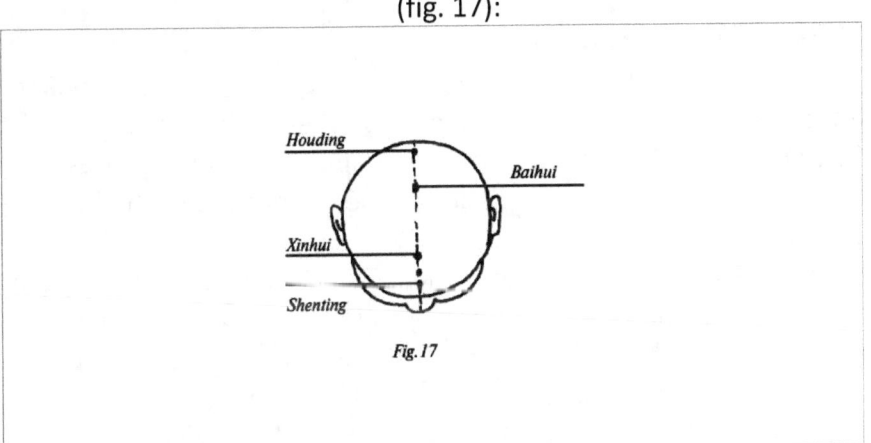

Fig. 17

Houding – GV19 (The back top) is located on the midline of the head, thirteen centimeters above the back hairline.

Baihui – GV20(The hundred meetings) is located on the midline of the head, at a distance of about seventeen centimeters from the back hairline and at a distance of about twelve centimeters from the front hairline. Sometimes the point is determined by the middle of the line, connecting the top of the ears.

Qianding – GV21 (The front hill) is located on the midline of the head, seven centimeters above the Shentin point (fig. 17).

Xinhui – GV22 (The compound of the skull) is located at the midline of the head, approximately five centimeters above the front hairline.

Shenting – GV24 (The yard of the spirit) (fig. 17).

Acupuncture points on the back of the head
(fig. 18):

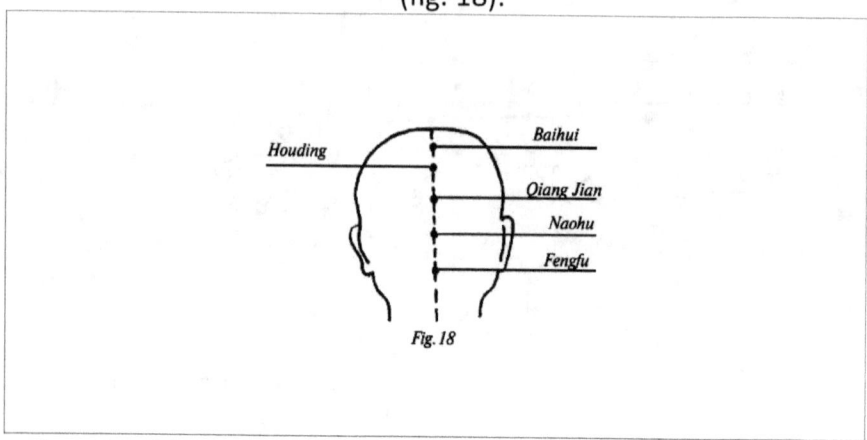

Fig. 18

Houding (The back top) (fig. 17).

Qiangjian – GV18 (The place of power) is located on the midline of the head, about ten centimeters above the hairline back.

Naohu – GV17 (The door of the brain) - the top "outpost" is located on the midline of thehead, on the upper edge of the back of the head.

Fengfu – GV16 (The palace of the wind) is located between the occipital bone and the 1st cervical vertebra, about tow centimeters above the back hairline. This point is the part of the intracranial pump, lifting up the spinal fluid and the flow of the Qi energy.

The acupuncture points,
which are located on the extremities:

Laogong – PC8 (The labor palace) is located in the center of the palm, in the gap between the tips of the 3rd and 4th fingers (fig. 19). This point refers to the Pericardium meridian.

Yongquan – KD1 (The boiling spring) is located on the bottom of the leg, on the third of the distance from a point between the base of the 2nd and 3rd toes to the heel end (Fig. 20). It is believed that the energy of the Earth passes through this point. The clearing of this energy before entering human energy system happens there. This point refers to the Kidney meridian.

Dadun – LV1 (The great revelation) is located on the lateral side of the rear tip of the big toe, 0,3 cm proximal to the corner of the nail (fig. 21).

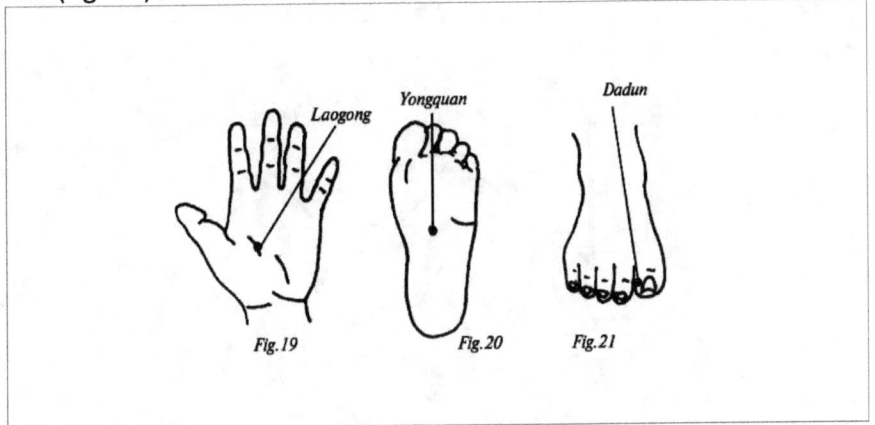

The acupuncture points
are located on the dorsal side of the body
(fig. 22):

Mingmen – GV4 (The gates of life) is located between the axis spurs of the 2nd and 3rd lumbar vertebrae. This point is the energy center of the kidneys and is the home to a congenital Qi.

The acupuncture points, located on the front of the body

(fig. 23):

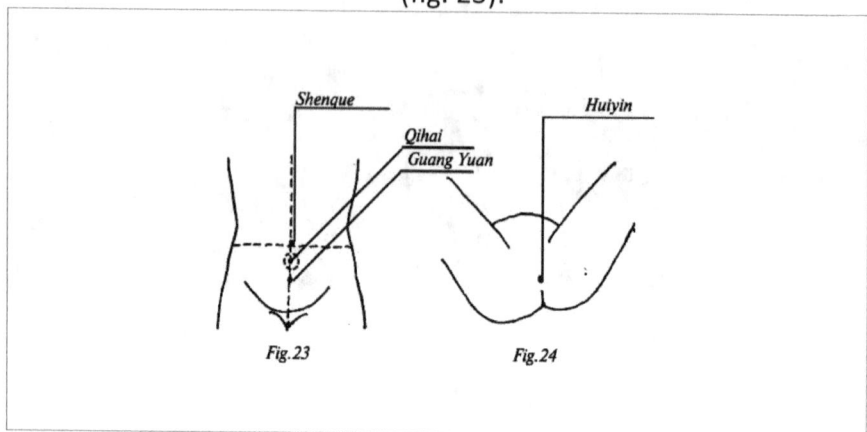

Fig.23   Fig.24

Shenque – CV8 (The place of the spirit) is located in the center of the navel. The navel - is the front door of the boiler (the lower Dantian), the place where the transformed various types of energies are mixed.

Qihai – CV6 (The sea of power) - the lower Dantian. It is located on the midline of the stomach, 4 centimeters below the belly button. The lower Dantien is the place where the Primary Qi and the energy converted into the life force are stored.

Guanyuan – CV4 (The projection point) is located on the middle line of the stomach, about seven and a half centimeters below the navel. The superficial epigastric lower artery, vein and the frontal dermal branches of the eleventh and twelfth intercostal nerves are situated in this area.

Huiying – CV1 (Merge of Yin) is located between the external genitals and the anus (fig.24) (between the anus and the scrotum to the males and posterior commissure of the labia majora to the women. This point is called the point of life and death. The energy pump which pushes the energy up through the spinal column, thus helping, the Qi to move along the microscopic orbit, is located in his area.

Dantians

In addition to the meridians a huge role in the regulation of the Qi energy flows play a specific areas, which are called **Dantian**. There is a significant concentration of Qi, and the processes of interaction of various kinds of energy in these points.

The three points are considered in Qigong:

1) The **Upper Dantian** - correspondence: top - point **Baihui** (top) and **Yintang** (between the eyebrows) from the front of the head (Fig. 15);

2) The **Medium Dantian** – is located in the solar plexus and corresponds to the point **Dan zhong** – CV15 (Fig. 25);

3) The **Lower Dantian** - is about 4 cm below the navel and corresponds to the point **Qihai** – CV6 (Fig. 25).

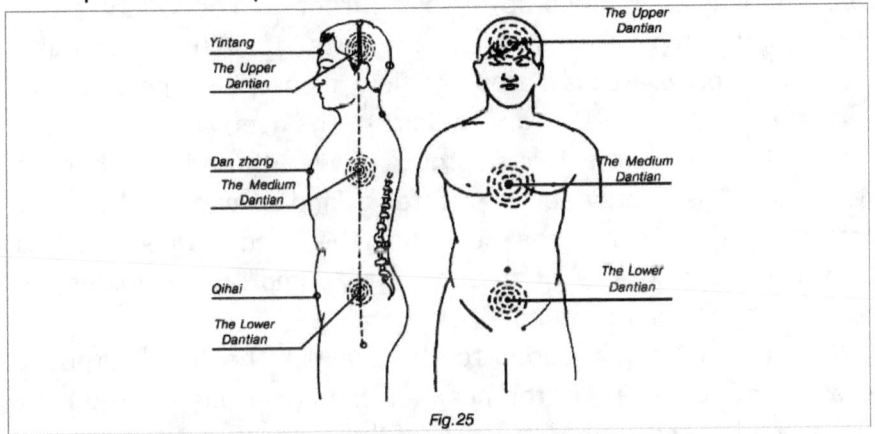

Fig.25

"Outposts"

The alternative to the three Dantians, are the three points, called **"Outposts"**. The flow of energy occurs with some difficulty in this points, and accordingly, to avoid the stagnation of the Qi, it is necessary to pay special attention to them. All the three gates are located on the Back-medium meridian (Du-mai) and are located at the following points: **Chang qiang** GV1, **Ling tai** – GV10 and **Naohu** – GV17 (Fig. 26).

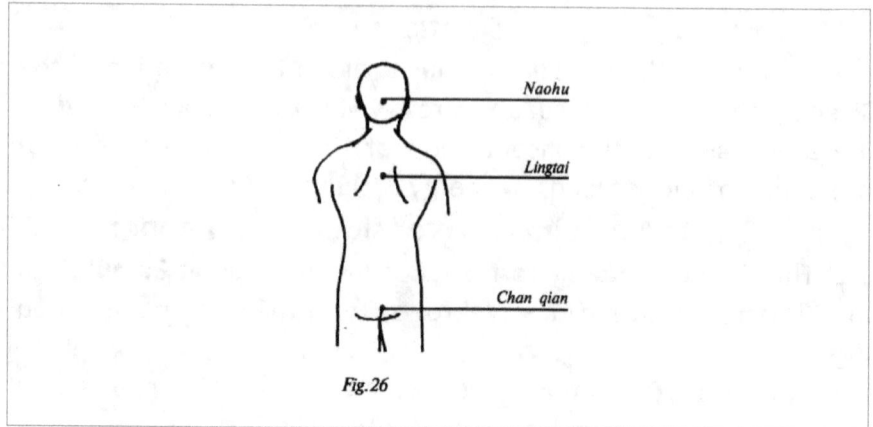

Fig. 26

Chang qiang – GV1 (The Rise of Force) - is the lower, "outpost", located midway between the tip of the coccyx and the anus. As the Qi energy begins to move up the spine from the coccyx, there is a close relationship between it and the lower Dantian. If for some reason the coccyx area is closed, the flow of energy will be blocked.

Lingtai – GV10 (The Terrace of Spirit) - the average "outpost", is located between the spinous sprouts of the 6th and 7th thoracic vertebrae. This energy center creates a kind of energy shell that protects the centers of the heart and the head. Sometimes this point is playing the role of an additional "pump" which guides the energy to the higher centers.

Naohu – GV17 (The Door to the Brain) - the top "outpost", located on the midline of the head, on the upper edge of the back of the head. In the energy structure of the human body, this point is considered to be the place where the flow of energy is particularly difficult.

Practicing Qigong it is necessary to study the localization and the main characteristics of the most frequently used energy points, the vast majority of which is located on Back-medium "Governing Vessel meridian" (Du Mai) and Frontal-medium "Conception Vessel meridian" (Ren Mai) meridians.

Chapter 1

The basic rules of Qigong

There are principles and rules the same in most schools and styles in Qigong. Since ancient times, these rules are called "The three important components of" Qigong ", which include:" **The Regulation of Consciousness "," The Regulation of Breathing** " and " **The Regulation of the Body**".

Any training is aimed to work with the internal energy Qi, and must be carried out strictly in accordance with these rules.

"The Regulation of Consciousness"

The regulation of consciousness - is the most important field of activity in Qigong, as all the activities, such as working out the positions and the rearrangement of breathing are trained under the guidance of consciousness. If you are unable to focus your attention, the talks about other practical techniques – are empty words. It is important to calm down, to eliminate extraneous thoughts, to concentrate on training activities and to sink into a state of rest during the training Qigong.

"The Regulation of Breathing"

The breathing process in the human body is controlled by the autonomic nervous system, so it can be controlled: consciously accelerate or slow down the pace of breathing, inhaling more deeply or do less.

There are several types of breathing used for certain manipulations with the movement of Qi energy in Qigong. Let's list the main types of breathing:

1) The natural breathing

The natural breathing is the breath when a person breathes the way he always used to do.

2) The deep breathing

The deep breathing is a variant of the natural breathing and is characterized by gradual lengthening of the exhalation and inhalation. Each subsequent respiratory action becomes longer. This process should be carried out naturally, without deliberate restraint of breath.

3) The belly breathing
(abdominal breathing)

This type of breathing is accomplished by a conscious protrusion and retraction of the belly, accompanying each inhalation and exhalation (Fig. 1).

4) The direct belly breathing

Direct belly breathing (the direct abdominal breathing) is carried out in such a way that while inhaling the belly bulges out smoothly, and on the exhale - feed (Fig. 2-4).

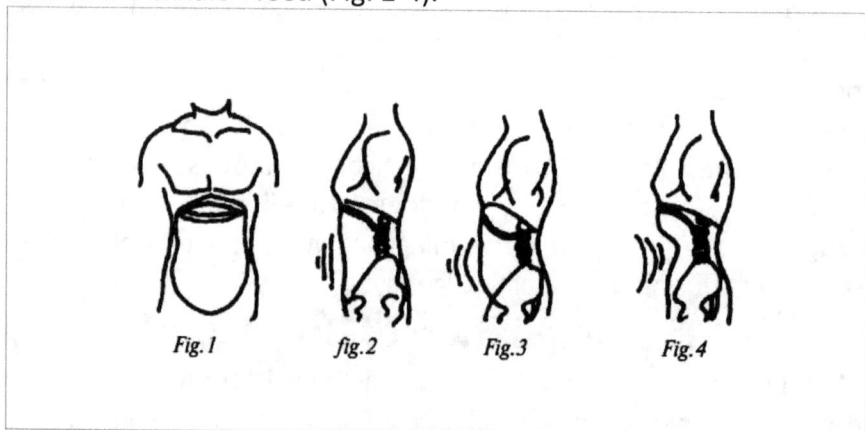

Fig. 1   fig.2   Fig.3   Fig.4

5) The reverse belly breathing

The reverse abdominal breathing is produced by the fact that during inhalation the belly retracts smoothly, and as you exhale - bulges (Fig. 5-7).

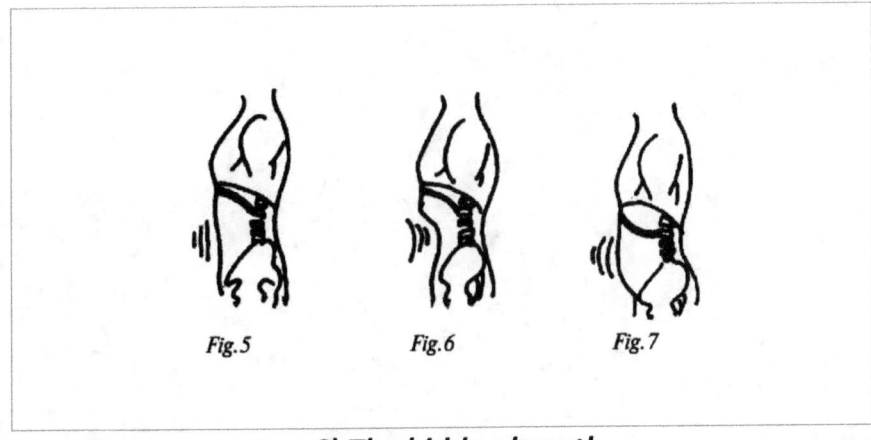

Fig.5   Fig.6   Fig.7

6) The hidden breath

The hidden breathing is done by raising and lowering of the lower part of the belly, which is achieved by carrying out a very soft exhalations and inhalations.

7) The umbilical (embryonic) breath

The umbilical breath - this is the most soft belly breathing, during which the belly almost is not moving. It is necessary to imagine that the navel area is breathing.

8) The breathing with pulling the anus

Draw consciously in the merge area Yin (point Huiyin) on the inhale, and let it go down on the exhale.

"The regulation of the body"

During the practice of Qigong it is required that all parts of the body are in their natural physiological conditions. The attention of the training person is focused on relaxation of the whole body and correction of breathing. By taking the correct position, the circulation of Qi through the channels and blood vessels improves. The basic requirements are: "Relaxation", "Peace" and "Nature."

Before the training Qigong it is important to achieve the state of relaxation that allows you to enter into a state of complete concentration. There is a special form which allows the body to relax "through the three lines" (Fig. 8, 9).

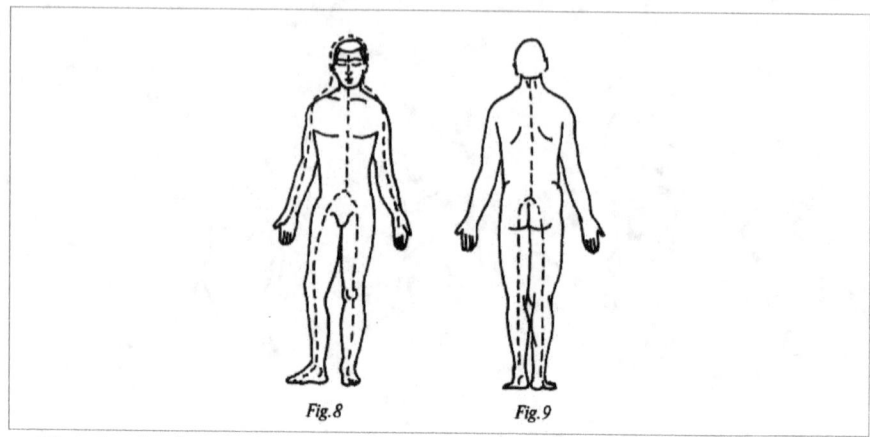

Fig. 8   Fig. 9

The body is conventionally divided down with a few lines on which the relaxation is produced in turn.

The first line of relaxation:

The sides of the head and neck - shoulders - upper arms - elbows - forearms - wrists - hands - ten fingers.

The second line of relaxation:

Face - neck - chest - belly - hips - knees - legs - feet - ten fingers.

The third line of relaxation:

Back of the head - the back of the neck - back - waist - back of the hips - basins under the knees - legs - feet - soles.

The relaxation is made in this sequence involving breathing. Take a deep breath in through your mouth. On the exhale, relax the relevant part of the body. The relaxation of each part is performed three times together.

For further practice of Qigong it is important to know the basic requirements of the position of the various parts of the body.

1. The head

The head should be kept straight. It seemes to be hang on the Baihui point. The chin tucked up a little.

2. The tounge

The tip of the tongue easily stretches into the upper palate (Fig. 10). Squeeze the teeth lightly. This is made to connect the Frontal-medium and the Backward-medium meridians, which occurs at the contact place of the tongue and palate.

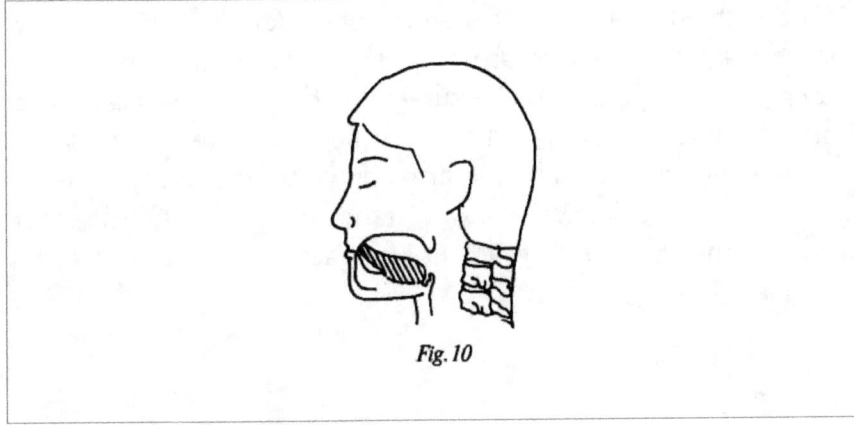

Fig. 10

3. The back and chest
The back should be straight and the chest retracted slightly.

4. The hands
The shoulders should be lowered and relaxed, hang over your elbows, hands - completely relaxed.

5. The loin
The loin should be relaxed and lowered a little.

6. The perineum
The perineum and anus need a little pull.

7. The feet
The knees are slightly bent. The toes as if raking the ground, the point Youngqyuan,
located on the feet, are slightly elevated.

On the next step, you need to master the **basic positions** to practice Qigong.

All positions are divided into the three big categories:
- *The standing position;*
- *The sitting position;*
- *The lying position;*

The standing position
There are several varieties of the standing position, they differ only by the hand position, the degree of bending of the knees and the width of the spaced legs. Let's describe the basic stance, which is the basis for the other taking positions in this category.

Stand with your feet wider than the shoulder width and slightly bend your knees. The feet are parallel to each other, the fingers "resting" on the ground. Make sure that the back is straight. The points Baihui (the crown) and Huiyin (the groin) are on the same imaginary vertical line. Take the arms down to your sides – to the sides so that the palms were at a distance of about two fists from your hips. The palms facing down. The gaze is directed forward - down (Fig. 11).

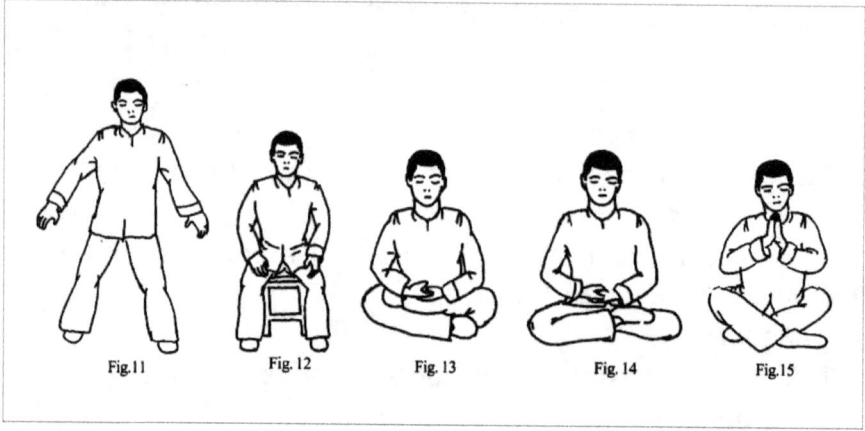

Fig.11   Fig. 12   Fig. 13   Fig. 14   Fig.15

The sitting position

Most of the activities "The circulation of Qi" and the meditative practices are trained in the positions of this category. Most of these positions are interchangeable and differ in their degree of acceptance.

The position of sitting on a stool

Sit down on a stool or a wooden chair. The back should not touch the back of the chair. Keep the head and torso upright and naturally. The back is straight, the points Baihui (the crown) and Huiyin (the groin) should be on the same imaginary vertical line. The feet are parallel to each other and completely touching the ground. The knees are bent, the angle between the hips and the lower leg should be about 90°. Take your hands on your hips, the palms centers are facing down, the fingers are facing forward (Fig. 12).

The half lotus

Sit down on the floor, on the rug, bed or specially reserved place for this purpose. Bend your knees. The foot of one leg lay on the inner part of the hip of the other leg. Keep your back straight. Put your hands on one another in front of the lower part of the belly. The palms are facing upward, the thumb is brushed aside. You can put both palms on the hips (Fig. 13).

The lotus

Sit on the floor or other smooth surface. Bend your knees. Turn the feet of both legs soles up and put them on the hips of each other. Straighten your back. Put your hands on one another in front of the lower part of the belly. The palms are facing upwards, the thumb is brushed aside. You can put both palms on the hips (Fig. 14).

The position with the crossed legs

Sit down on the floor or other smooth surface. Bend your knees and cross your legs. Keep your back straight. The hands are either in the described above positions, or in the position of prayer (Fig. 15).

The lying positions

The lying on the back position

Lie down on the floor or other smooth surface on the back. Stretch horizontally. Put your head on the pillow so that the neck was in an upright position. Close your eyes and mouth. The back should be straight. Bend your elbows and place them behind your head. You can place the hands one above the other on your belly, with your hands to the center of the belly (Fig. 16).

The position of lying on your side

Lie down on the floor or other smooth surface on the right side. Close your eyes. The tip of the tongue rests against the upper palate. Place the right hand on the pillow under your head. Put the left hand along the side. The left leg is slightly bent at the knee (Fig. 17).

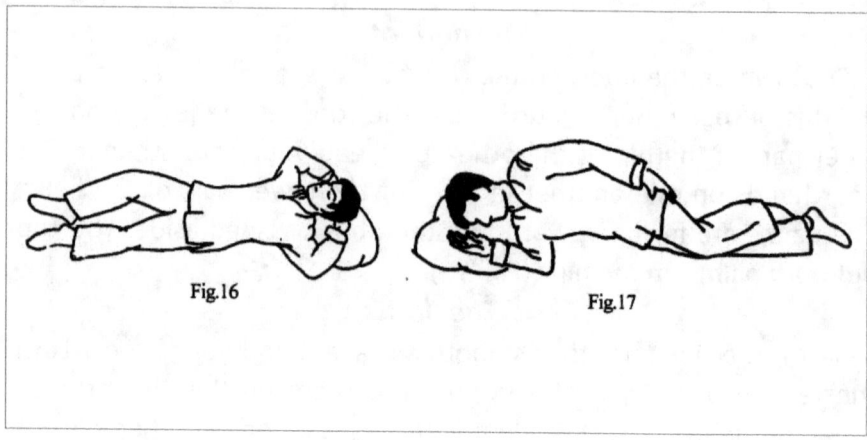

Fig.16   Fig.17

Chapter 2
Theoretical Aspects of the Tianzhu Shan Qigong system

Tianzhu Shan Qigong system is a kind of the ancient **Daoist «Art of Inner pill"**. The concept of "inner pill" - is the antagonism of the notion "Outer pill." Medieval alchemists tried to develop a formula of some medicine (pill) in searches of ways to achieve immortality, taking of which could lead to the desired effect. This medicine was called "Outer pill". It was produced by melting of lead, mercury and other ingredients in special chemical crucibles on a tripod. It is known that few very important people, among who were even the emperors of China, after taking such a drug were died in agony. Accordingly, "The Art of outer pill" had fallen into disrepair and disappeared.

Despite the almost complete disappearance, the terminology of this art was inherited by the replaced it art of the "Inner alchemy". Here, the "pill of immortality" is prepared inside the human body of the ingredients such as: **Seed-Jing**, **Qi** and **Spirit-Shen**. Herein as the alchemical tripod is used the human body, bellows to force the air - Spirit-Shen, and the air, blowing the fire - Qi, obtained during the breathing.

Seed-Jing – is a substance that forms the human body and the underlying is the base of functioning of all its systems. Jing is of two kinds: **"Pre Heaven"**, obtained from the parents and the **"Post Heaven"**, extracted from the food. The storage place of the "Post Heaven" Jing are the kidneys. In the theory of the "Inner" alchemy, Seed-Jing is considered a basic component of the **"Inner pill"**.

Qi - is the energy substance, forming the world. All the things, processes and phenomena in the Universe are due to the movement and transformation of Qi. In the human body Qi plays the role of the driving force of birth, growth and development, as well as thanks to its metabolic processes occur. Qi is divided into "original", "main", "feeding", "protective" etc. The "Original» Qi is classified as "Pre Celestial" and is an important substance in the practice of Qigong. "Main" Qi, «Feeding» Qi and "Protective" Qi are classified as "Post Heaven" and provide the heart work, breathing, nutrition and immune system of the organism. In theory of the "Inner" alchemy the "Pre Heaven" Qi is one of the main ingredients in the preparation of the "Immortality pill" and the "Post Celestial" Qi fulfills the function of heating and power.

Spirit-Shen - is the ultimate manifestation of vital activity of the organism, consciousness and thinking, and serves as a control function. In theory of the "Inner" alchemy, Spirit-Shen and thought is the third of the fundamental components of the "pill".

It is believed that Jing, Qi and Shen can be converted into each other and have a common term for their determnation - "Three Jewels".

In the Tianzhu Shan Qigong system the three types of action "Three Jewels" are produced:
- *"Calming the mind to cultivate the seed" to avoid the Seed, Qi and Spirit dispersal.*
- *"Concentration on the single".*
- *"Gathering of the Qi». There the Qi of Heaven, Earth and Man mix and the enrichment of the "Substance of pill".*

The melting process of the **"Inner pill of immortality"** is divided into four stages: **"Laying the foundation"**, **"Mixing Jing, Qi and Shen»**, **«Melting the Spirit out of Qi»**, **«Melting the Spirit and returning to the eptiness"**.

"Laying the foundations" - is primarily a training of the body for all subsequent practices: getting rid of diseases, restoration of the disturbed functions of the organism, restocking of the Seed-Jing, Qi and Spirit-Shen. This stage is completed during the practice of the dynamic exercises, when as a result of exercises enough of "Drugs" accumulate and the cleaning of meridians appears.

"Mixing of Jing, Qi and Shen" - is the second stage of "Overcoming of the initial outpost". It completes after a 36-day job of concentration on the lower Dantian Qi and moving of Qi on the "Small heaven circle". On the "Small Heaven Circle" the Spirit and the thought lead the Qi with the aim of melting the pill. The movement of the energy is carried out along two wonderful meridians Du-mai and Ren-mai.

"Melting of Spirit of Qi" - is the third stage ("Overcoming the average outpost") in the practice of melting of "Immortality pill". There is moving of Qi between the Middle and Lower Dantians here. After 36 days «Qi pill" will be freely moving along this way, or even along the "Great heaven circle". The motion of energy along the "Great heaven circle" is made along all eight wonderful meridians. If to carry Qi on this route hard, one of the fundamental principles of Qigong of «Relaxation and tranquility" will be broken. Therefore, to ensure the circulation of Qi through the remaining six "Wonderful" meridians, except Ren-mai and Du-mai and through the twelve "main" channels a great care of concentration is not required. It is enough simply to clarify the route and the process of moving of energy in general. By the time of circulation through the "large celestial circle" the "Golden Pill" is already formed, the free patency of all energy channels s provided. Thus, the "pill" circulates spontaneously, without active mental "leading" it through the route. Accordingly, there is no need to focus on it.

"Melting the Spirit and return to the emptiness" - is the fourth final stage of "Inner Alchemy", it was earlier considered to be confidential. The enlightenment, "clearing the heart", "epiphany of truth" and the possibility of reaching a state of immortality occur here.

Another term is **"Tripod and oven"** - a concept that is interpreted differently in different schools of Qigong. In the Tianzhu Shan Qigong system at the first stage ("Overcoming of initial outposts") the "Tripod" - is the upward Dantian, and the "Oven" - is the lower Dantian. The system of mutual work is called "Great tripod and oven". At this stage the focusing on the lower Dantian drives «Qi pill", which starts to circulate along the Ren-mai and Du-mai meridians.

In the stage of " **Overcoming of initial outposts"** the "Tripod" is considered the average Dantian, and the "Oven" – is the lower Dantian. Together they are called "Small tripod and oven". Here, the concentration is made on the average Dantian, implying that in the crucible of the tripod is formed the "drug" already, which must undergo the further melting, circulating between the awerage and lower Dantians. With this, the concentration should not be too strong, it is enough to focus on the idea of the "tripod and oven" in general.

There is an important concept **"Fire Environment"** in Qigong, which is "Spirit and thought", as well as the inhale and exhale Qi. Spirit - is "Fire", and breath – is "Wind". Leading the «Qi pill" along the Ren-mai meridian during inhale is called "movement of Yang fire», and the return of «Qi pill" to the area of the lower Dantian at the exhale is called "retreat under the Yin sign».

While **"gathering the Qi pill"** it is important to use the "Humane Fire", where the degree of attention is blurred a little and the inhale and exhale – are soft and smooth. When it is needed to move the "Golden pill" through the celestial circle to increase the number of "Spiritual Qi», they use the "militant fire" which represents a "Hot" mode of "Melting" Concentration of attention and breathing become more intense.

In the **Tianzhushan Qigong** system the gathering of Qi Heaven, Earth and "Ten thousand of things" replenishes Jing, Qi and Shen of a person and merge into "drug", which has a considerable energy. This speeds up the process of "ripening of pill". Leading it through the system of channels improves the throughput and eliminates the "plugs", prepares the conditions for "Plotting of pill" and its pass through the celestial circle. This provides a more rapid result comparing to other conventional techniques. Thus the Tianzhushan Qigong system reveals the secrets of the ancient Daoist «Inner Alchemy" and allows to move efficiently and quickly through the way of preparation of mysterious "Inner pill of immortality".

Chapter 3
Dynamic Qigong exercises

In the old days the Dynamic exercises were known as Daoin-shu - «The art of leading and attracting (of energy)". All the exercises in this section are characterized by a close interaction. So "Gathering of Qi», «Outmelting of pill" and "Movement through the" Celestial circle "are made simultaneously. It is important to watch the concentration of attention, shifting of the center of attention, movement and breathing were made, in a close coordination. In complexes and exercises is usually used the reverse abdominal breathing.

At a certain stage of training, the dynamic exercises can be combined with the static exercises, this increases their efficiency and effectiveness.

Section 1
"The art of taking of position of internal pill growing"

1. Starting position. Stand facing the South or East. Feet are together, knees are straightened, the feet toes as if "capture" the land, arms are extended down at the sides, head is straight, Bai Hui point, located at the crown is directed vertically upwards. Eyes are tightly covered (Fig. 1).

Slowly apply the hands palms on the stomach. Men put their right hand on the left hand, women on the contrary left hand is placed on the right hand. Laogong point, located in the center of the palms is located opposite to the Qihai point (approximately 4 cm below the navel). Laogong points of both hands should be projected at each other. With the tip of the tongue touch the sky behind the alveoli. Teeth are closed not very strongly. Shoulders and elbows are omitted. Legs are slightly bend at the knees (Fig. 2).

2. Keeping a smooth and calm rhythm, make from three to nine breaths cycles (inhale - exhale). Use the reverse abdominal type of breathing.

3. With a rotational motion of the hips make one turnover in the horizontal plane in a counterclockwise direction (Fig. 3).

4. With the left leg make a small step to the left. Rotating the hips make one turn in the horizontal plane in the clockwise direction. Fix the position standing up straight and slightly bending your knees (Fig. 4). This stance is called "Growing up the initial pill position".

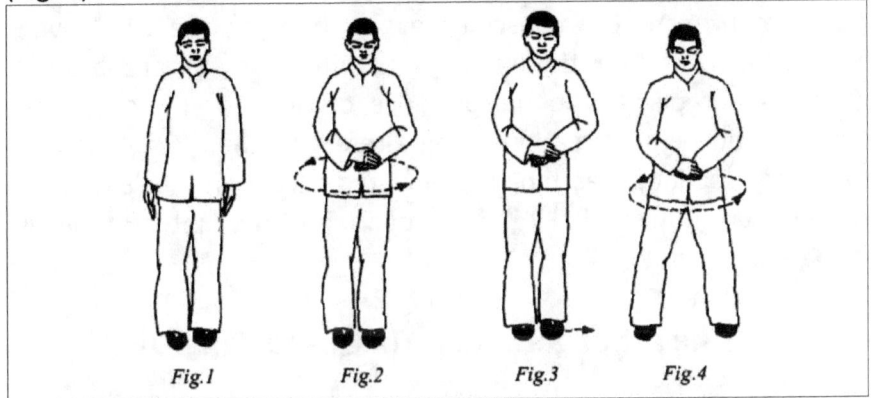

Fig.1   Fig.2   Fig.3   Fig.4

5. Being in the taken position make nine, thirty six, or one hundred eight breathing cycles using the reverse abdominal type of breathing.

Important points:

1. Orientation by sides of the world:
- From 23-00 to 11-00 - the face is directed to the East,
- From 11-00 to 23-00 - the face is directed to the South.

2. Hip rotation is made slowly without jerks and accelerations through a full circle. Knees operate as a kind of rotary axes.

3. Consciousness is focused on the performed actions.

4. During the rotation of the hips an association with a round "Celestial sphere" and the merge with the whole universe should appear.

"The art of taking the position of growing of the internal pill" is a preparation for the implementation of almost all major exercises and allows you to enter the so-called "State of Qigong».

This exercise can be performed separately as an independent complex.

Explanations:

"The art of taking the position of growing of the internal pill" is the basis for all dynamic Tianzhu Shan Qigong system exercises. Requirements which relate to the position and movements of the hips refer to the "Regulating of the body" section. Associations of the rotation of the hips with the circumference of the "Celestial sphere" refer to the "Regulating of consciousness" section. Here the task is to prepare the consciousness to bringing the Qi Heaven energy, Earth and "Ten thousand things to the body for preparation of the "Inner pill ". The performance of nine (or more to one hundred and eight) breathing cycles refers to the "Regulation of breathing" section. Breathing is associated here with the "Bellows". By which the power of "Fire" for preparing of the "Internal pill" is regulated.

Section 2
"The art of gathering Yin Qi and Yang Qi"

"Gathering of Qi (Yin) of the Earth"

1. Take the position of "Growing of the internal pill" (Fig. 5).

2. Turning the hands with palms directed forward, slowly lower your arms down. Make an exhale (Fig. 6).

3. Slowly rise up both hands in front of you to the shoulder level. Hands remain straightened at elbows. Make the breath. You as if pick up the "Earth Qi» and collect it with the palms (Fig. 7).

4. Bend your hands at elbows. The elbows are lowered. The forearms take a vertical position. Turning both hands with palms to you, with the circular motion move them to the chest. You as if enfold a big ball and move it to the chest. Take a breath (Fig. 8).

5. With a slow movement lower both hands down, putting the hands at each other. With your hands you as if with a gentle pressure lower Qi to the area of the lower Dantian. The Laogong points on the palms are situated opposite the Qihai point (approximately 4 cm below the navel). Take the breath (Fig. 9). Make the whole exercise three times.

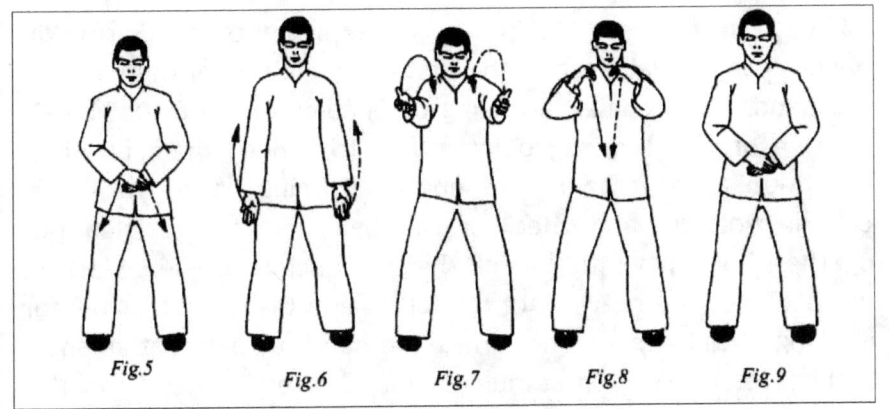

Fig.5   Fig.6   Fig.7   Fig.8   Fig.9

Important points:

1. During the "raising of Qi upward" it is necessary to liberate the forearms and focus the attention on the Laogong points, located in the center of the palms.

2. During the lowering of arms, the "pushing" movement by the brush should be made at some angle to the area of the average Dantian. This encourages the submergence of Qi therein.

3. When the palms take a position parallel to the Dantian area and pass down, Qi as if is pushed into it.

4. During the exercise, imagine that you are surrounded by warm Earth Qi energy which has the inexhaustible power which it gives to you.

Explanations:

In the art of "Inner Alchemy" it is believed that the Yang substances relate to the Sky and Yin – to the Earth. Sky and Earth - are the transformations of "Seed-Jing», «Celestial Yang» and «Earth Yin». Therefore, the primary task is gathering of energy Yang-Sky and Yin-Earth energies from the expanse of the surrounding world for the subsequent melting of the "Internal pill".

Since Yang "relies" on Yin and complements it, "Earth Yin substances» are gathered in the first place. Raising of the Earth Qi with hands should cause a feeling of "leading of the Qi upwards". Focusing on the Laogong points allow to "open" them for their perception and "gathering" of energy. Turning of the forearms, "covering of Qi» and "necking the ball" must be carried out together. This allows to "open" the acupuncture points, which in turn activates the network of meridians and the bone marrow for uptaking of Qi by them. The turn of the hands by palms at an angle to the average Dantian stimulates the "immersion" of Qi in this area. When the palms are parallel to Dantian and Qi «pressed into it", the sense of presence of energy becomes more distinct.

"Gathering of the celestial (Yang) Qi»

This exercise is a continuation of the previous one.

1. From the starting position of "Growing of the internal pill" make three breathing cycles (inhale-exhale) (Fig. 10).

2. With a slow movement expand hand with palms up and move them to the sides of the torso. At the same time, make an exhale (Fig. 11).

3. Moving the hand along the frontal sides of the torso, lift them up to the level of the average Dantian. Simultaneously make an inhale (Fig. 12).

4. Move your elbows forward and down. Forearms are arranged vertically, palms are facing you. Hands are at a distance of about 30 centimeters from the chest. You as if support by the hands a large bowl. At the same time, make an inhale (Fig. 13).

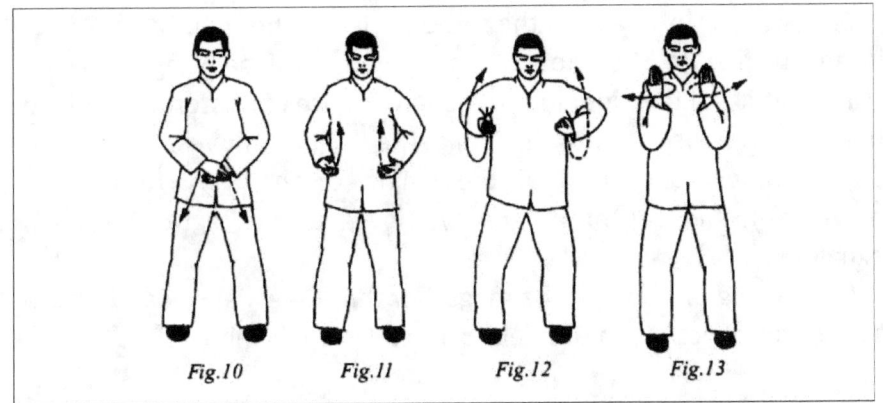

Fig.10   Fig.11   Fig.12   Fig.13

5. Using elbows as the center of rotation, move hands to the sides on an arc. Palms are angled upwards (Fig. 14).

6. Hold the right hand stationary. The left hand moves in an arc first to shoulder, and then, as if painting a sign of "Great limit" (Taiji) to the side. In the movement are consistently involved the elbow, wrist and fingers. The hand moves aside for approximately one third of the length of the arm. During the movement, the center of gravity shifts to the left. Simultaneously make an exhale (Fig. 15).

7. Focusing on the left hand, gather "The celestial Qi» and return it to the center of gravity in the flat position. Simultaneously make an inhale (Fig. 16).

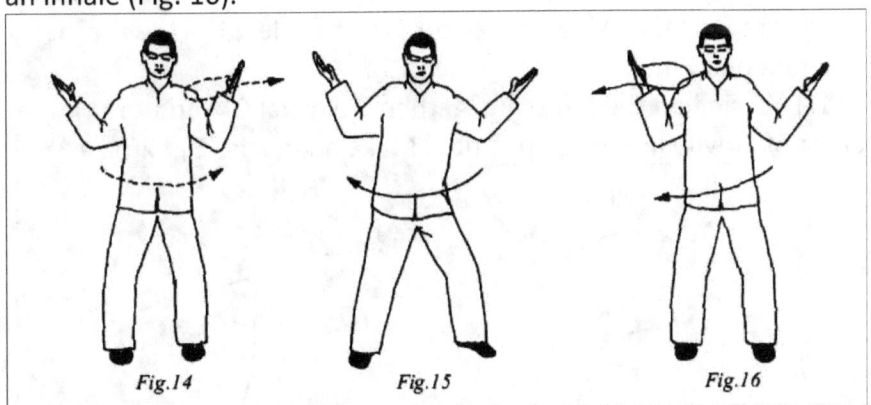

Fig.14   Fig.15   Fig.16

8. Hold your left hand in the same position. The right hand moves in an arc first to the shoulder, and then, as if painting a sign of "Great limit" to the side. In the movement are consistently involved the elbow, wrist and fingers. The hand moves aside for approximately one third of the length of the arm. During the movement, the center of gravity moves to the right. Make an exhale (Fig. 17).

9. Focusing on the right palm, gather the "Celestial Qi» and return the center of gravity in the flat position. Make an inhale (Fig. 18).

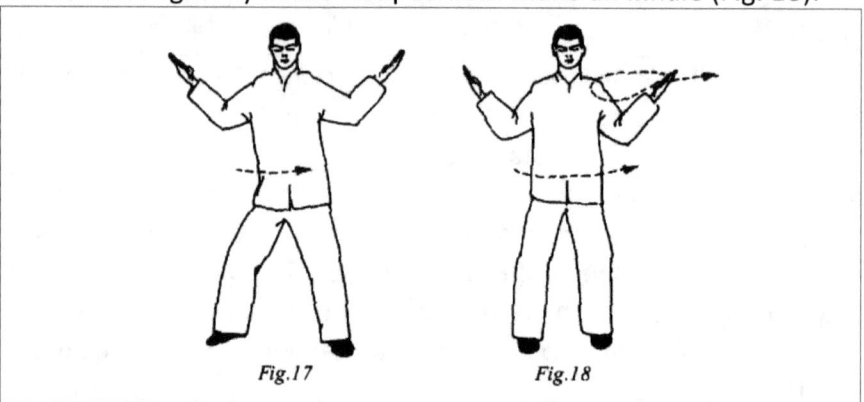

Fig.17   Fig.18

10. Shift the center of gravity to the left. Hold the right hand stationary. Similarly, with a movement from the shoulder, including into it consistently the elbow, wrist and fingers move the left hand in an arc to the side by one-third the length to the left. Simultaneously make an exhale (Fig. 19).

11. Focusing on the left palm, gather "Celestial Qi» and return the center of gravity in the flat position. Make an inhale (Fig. 20).

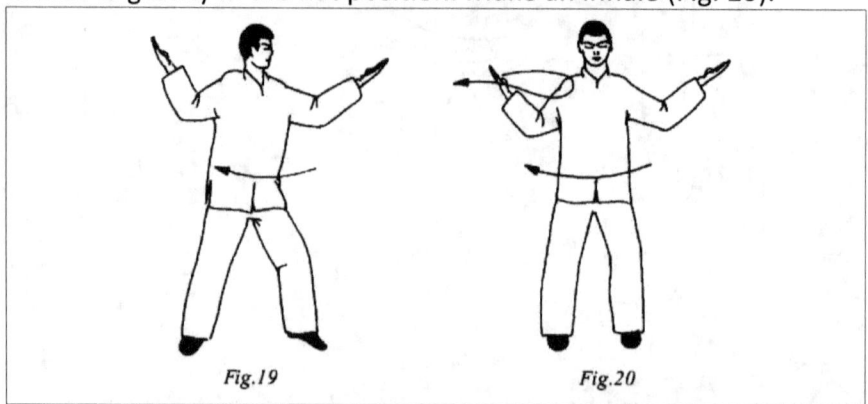

Fig.19   Fig.20

12. Shift the center of gravity to the right. Hold the left hand stationary. With a movement from the shoulder, including the elbow, wrist and fingers, move the right hand in an arc to the side at one-third the length to the right. Simultaneously make an exhale (Fig. 21).

13. Focusing on the right palm, gather "Celestial Qi" and return the center of gravity in the flat position. Make an inhale (Fig. 22).

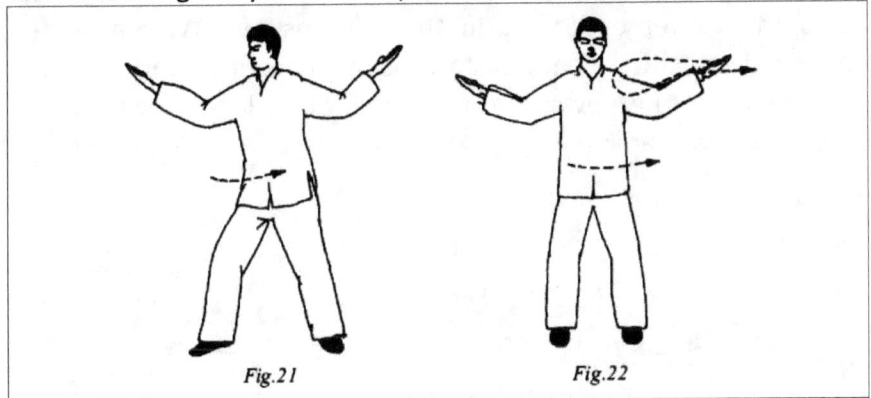

Fig.21   Fig.22

14. Shift the center of gravity to the left. Hold the right hand stationary. With a movement from the shoulder including the elbow, wrist and fingers, move the left hand in an arc to the side at the last third to the left.

Unlike the previous movements it is important to raise the hand from the shoulder joint to the elbow in an arc upwards a little. Simultaneously make an exhale (Fig. 23).

15. Focusing on the left hand, gather the "Celestial Qi» and return the center of gravity to the flat position. Make an inhale (Fig. 24).

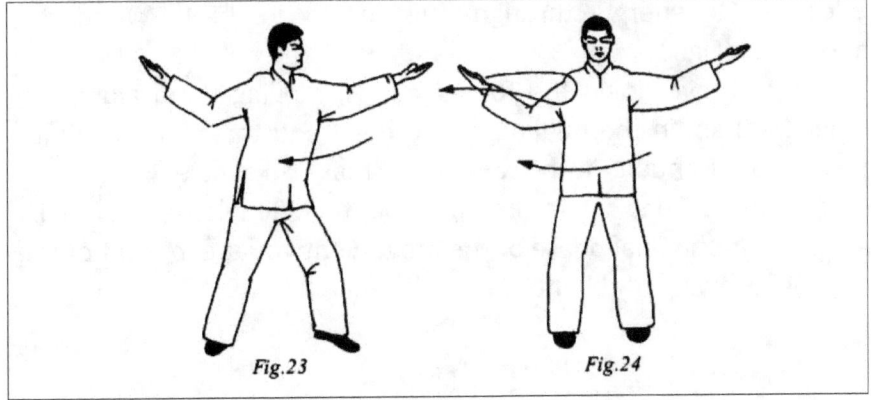

Fig.23   Fig.24

16. Shift the center of gravity to the right. Hold the left hand stationary. With the movement from the shoulder including the elbow, wrist and fingers, move the right hand in an arc to the side at the last third of the length to the right. It is necessary to raise the hand from the shoulder joint to the elbow in an arc upwards a little. Simultaneously make an exhale (Fig. 25).

17. Focusing on the right palm, gather the "Celestial Qi» and return the center of gravity in the flat position. With a gentle movement of the forearms start as if "covering" the Qi. The forearms are rising upward. You as if enfold a large bowl. At the same time, make an inhale (Fig. 26).

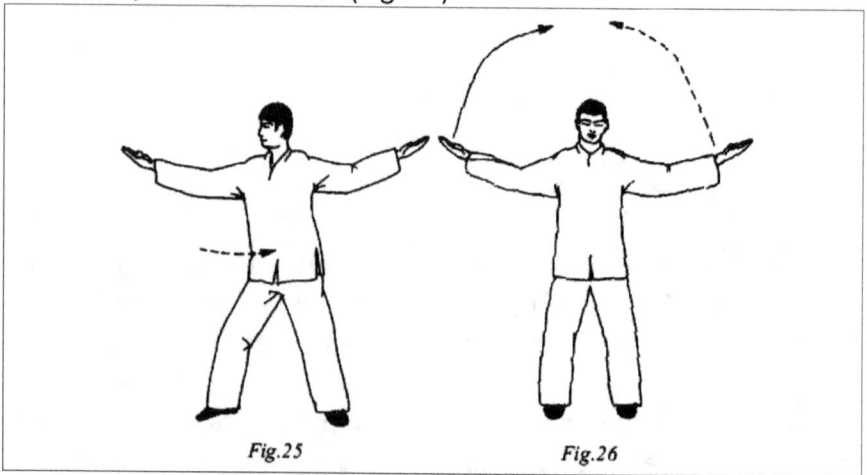

Fig.25   Fig.26

18. Continuing to "enfold" Qi over the head, put the hands on each other by joining the projections of Laogong points and turning them toward the Baihui point, located on the crown. You "press" collected Qi energy through this point in "The Wonderful meridians" (Fig. 27).

Start to move down the folded hands, moving them along the upper Dantian, in the midline of the head and torso. "Lead" Qi to the medium Dantian. At the same time, make an exhale (Fig. 28).

Continue to "lead" Qi to the lower Dantian. Simultaneously make an inhale. In the final phase of the movement you are in front of the original "Growing of the internal pill" stance (Fig. 29).

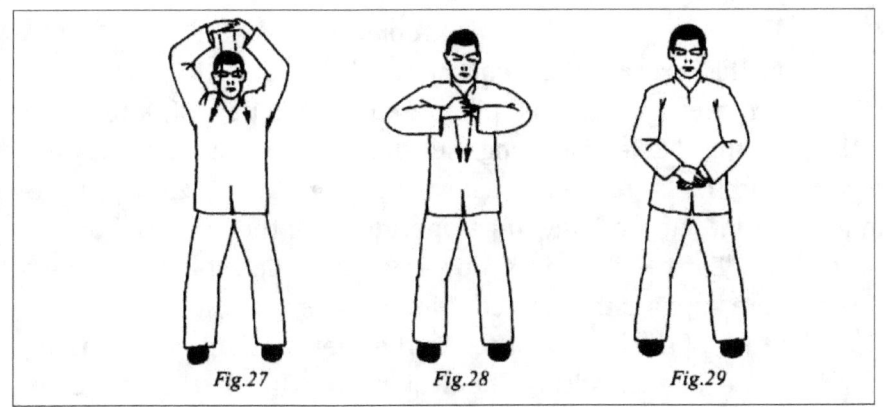

Fig.27   Fig.28   Fig.29

Important points:

1. Moving hands to the sides of the body, moving them up and "rising ball" in front of you, you involve the "Earth Qi (Yin)" in cooperation with the "Celestial Qi (Yang)".

2. Phased moving arms to the sides, move the center of gravity of the body in the same direction, where the hand moves.

3. During the movement of the hand to the side the movement of Qi to the finger-tips is felt, however it is not necessary to lead mentally the energy outside the extremities and body.

4. When the aside movement of the hand finishes and the stream of Qi comes to the fingers, at the same time make an inhale and "Gathering of the Celestial Qi". Attention is carried to space. There is a feeling of "catching" of Qi in palms. At this time the Centre of gravity of the body becomes straight.

5. In the moment of "hugging the bawl" attention moves out in space again in an order to lead the "Celestial Qi (Yang)" to the Baihui point.

6. Further the energy moves downward on the frontal-medium Ren - mai meridian and "submerges" in the lower Dantian, here must be the sense of "penetration" of the energy in this area.

Explanations:

Making this exercise you collect the "Celestial Qi (Yang)" as a component for an internal pill. Among all types of energy of Universe, the "Celestial Yang substances" are considered the hardest and the largest ones. Celestial Qi is motive force which sets in motion and, accordingly in co-operation, all the forces of Space. When the "Earth Qi" moves upwards, and "Celestial Qi" lowers down, there appears the "Mixed Primordial Qi".

At the turn of the hands turned to the average Dantian, palms up, moved aside hands, raising them along the front sides of torso, forward movement of the hands, moving aside of hands and raising them upwards, is necessary to imagine that the "Earth Qi" is joined with the "Celestial Qi". Moving of center of the focusing and movement must have a continuous process.

It is necessary for the Yang-substances could join with Yin-substances and get into the body. During the changeable movement of the arms to the sides it is necessary to imagine that the energetic channels "open" for the movement of energy through them. At the end of each aside movement of the arm, simultaneously with the inhale and shifting the gravity center to the starting point, gather Qi with the palms. When you "Raise Qi upwards", it is necessary to imagine Qi, dissolved in the endless space of the Universe. Qi is well-felt during the "Direction" of it to the Baihui point. When the energy is lead to the awerage Dantian, direct your gaze "inside yourself".

"Nine circulations of the energy in Dantian"

This exercise is the continuation of the previous one.

1. The starting position "Growing of the inner pill".

2. Mentally imagine that in the area of the lower Dantian is the "energy bawl".

3. Start with making soft and light circle movements, with put palm on the Dantian. The direction of the movement-counterclockwise (Fig. 30).

At each circle movement of palms should be one breathing cycle: half a circle-inhale, half a circle- exhale.

Thus, the make nine circle movements with palms.

3. Analogic to the described above example make nine circle movements with the palms in the other direction (Fig. 31).

4. Get back to the starting position of "Growing of the inner pill" (Fig. 32).

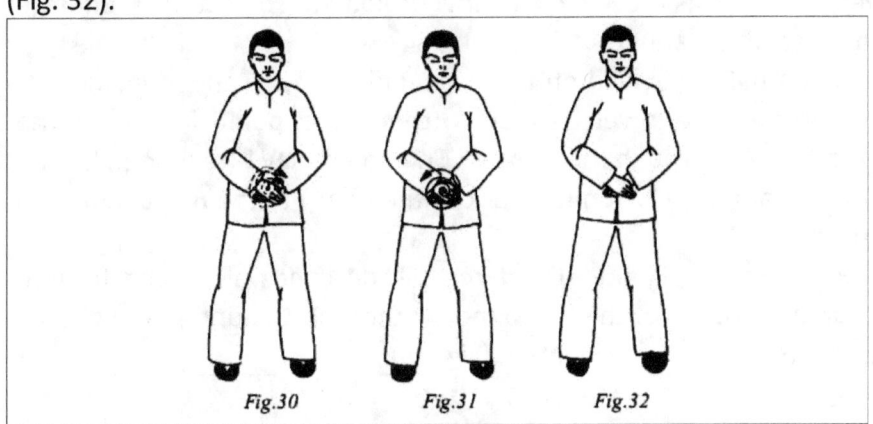

Fig.30   Fig.31   Fig.32

Important points:

1. It is necessary to imagine mentally a ball in the lower Dantien, wich consists of the Qi energy.

2. The circle movements with the palms should be accompanied with the feeling of the "circulation" of this concentration of energy.

Explanations:

Making tis exercise you join the Celestial, Earth and Human Qi energies into one substance in the lower Dantien. The gathered Celestial and Earth Qi energies mix with the seed-Jing, Qi and spirit-Shen of the man in some ingredient, the circulation of which in the area of Dantien leads to the appearance of the "Cureing ingredient". The circulation of this ingredient in the lower Dantien makes Qi of "three components" to join into the "Cure extract of the pill". In this moment at a very important place is the right breathing, which is the "wind" which blows the "fire" for melting the "pill". At the first stages of the "fire" power it must be enough for the "Heating and growing the Qi pill".

Some roundness of the palm is important for the fact that in the space under the palm there is some of Qi, necessary for "growing the pill". This exercise can be made by cycles by ten or thirty-six movements

"Movement through the celestial circle"

This exercise is the continuation of the previous one.

1. Starting position – stance of "Growing of the internal pill".

2. Make an inhale. Slowly pull in your belly and "lift the anus" very gently (this is achieved by low preload of sphincters - obdurate muscles of the anus).

« The pill Qi" is lead on the back-middle meridian (Du-mai) from the area of the lower Dantian to the Huiyin point, located in the crotch, then through the "gates": Chan qian - QV1 (tailbone), Lingtai QV10, Naohu GV17 (on the back of the head) to the Baihui point on the crown.

3. Make an exhale. «Qi of the pill descends along the frontal-middle meridian of the Baihui point, through the upper and middle Dantians to the lower Dantian (Fig. 33).

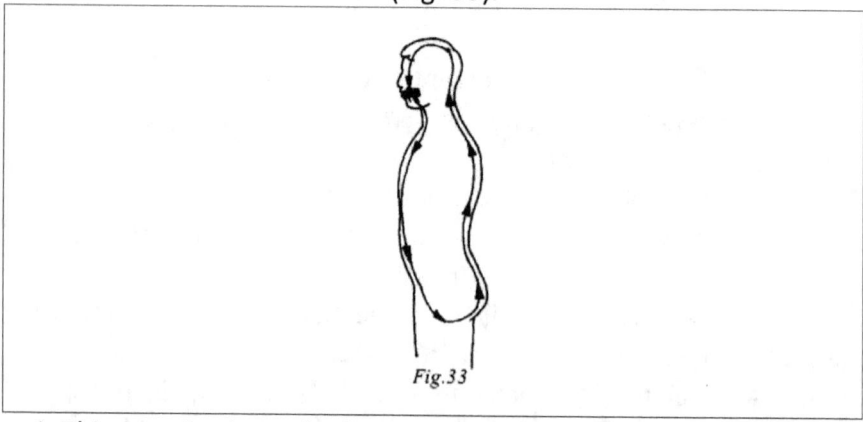

Fig.33

4. This exercise is made three or nine times.

Important points:

1. At an inhale the tip of the tongue is raised to the palate, at the exhale it moves down to the bottom of the palate.

2. Move up the area located between the last cervical and first thoracic vertebrae in order to "liberate" the back – middle meridian (Du-mai) for the unobstructed passage of Qi.

3. When Qi is moved to the back (barrier Naohu GV17) it is important to focus quickly on the Baihui point. This will be easier for the Qi energy to overcome this area.

4. After the exercise it is important just to breathe easy and literately for some time.

During making this exercise, you form a "Small Celestial Circle" and build circulation of Qi through it.

Explanations:

Du-mai meridian fulfills the work of "managing" the Qi actions of all meridians Yang, Ren-mai - Qi of all Yin meridians. These two "Wonderful" meridians supply twelve main meridians and other energy channels of Qi, accumulate it and regulate the activity of the entire network of meridians. "Circulating along the "Celestial circle "improves the patency of these two meridians, thereby make a regulating effect on the interaction of Yin and Yang substances in the human body, the quality of the functioning of the Qi and blood current through the main arteries and eliminate the dysfunctions in the work of the internal organs.

In the "Inner Alchemy" leading Qi through the thought on "Small Celestial Circle", involvement of the «Qi pill" into the circulation along it for further "melting", promotes the more rapid formation of the "Golden pill".

Thus, to summarize, we define three main stages in the Dynamic method of "melting of the inner pill". At the first stage the involved people collect Sky and Earth Qi to replenish inner stocks of "Seed, Qi and Spirit". At the second stage is the conversion of human, Earth and Sky Qi into "Curing ingredient", which through the means of nine circulations in Dantian area is processed and melted into the "Internal pill". At the third stage of the "Circulation through the celestial circle", "Curing ingredients" are further processed.

Section 3

"The opening of consciousness for a celestial mind"

1. Starting position – stance of "Growing of the internal pill" (Fig. 34).

2. At the exhale, lower your arms down, palms facing toward you (Fig.35).

3. At the inhale rotate the torso at the waist to the right. Move the left hand in front of you at shoulder level, the hand is turned up with the palm. Right hand palm down and moves under the left elbow at the waist level (Fig. 36).

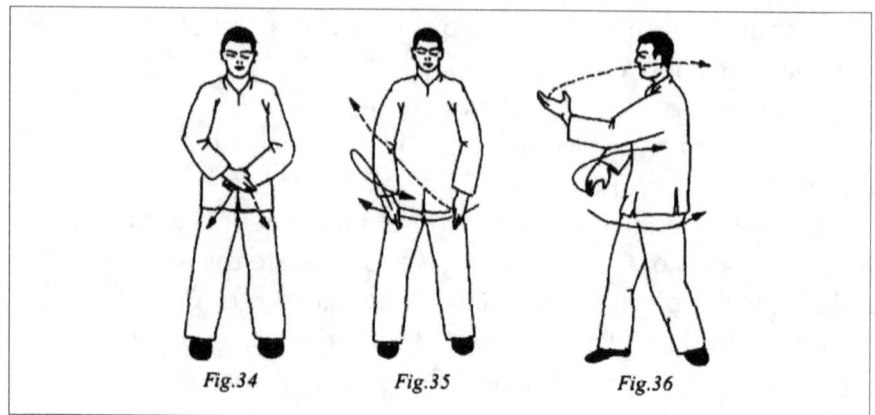

Fig.34   Fig.35   Fig.36

4. Continue to make the inhale. Hands do not change their position. Torso turns to the left. After that, just lift your hands up a little (Fig. 37).

5. Expand the left palm to the area of the upper Dantian. Move the hand from the trough, adjacent to the outer corner of the right eye, past the right shoulder, chest, right elbow, right lower part of abdomen to the left lower part of abdomen. At the same time, expand the right palm from you and make the movement of the forearm around the elbow on the circle to the right and down, then left and upwards. Torso turns to the right. Movement is made at an exhalation (Fig. 38).

6. At an inhale turn the torso at the waist to the left. Move the right hand in front of you at the shoulder level, palm turns up. Left hand turns with the palm down and is brought under the right elbow at the waist level (Fig. 39).

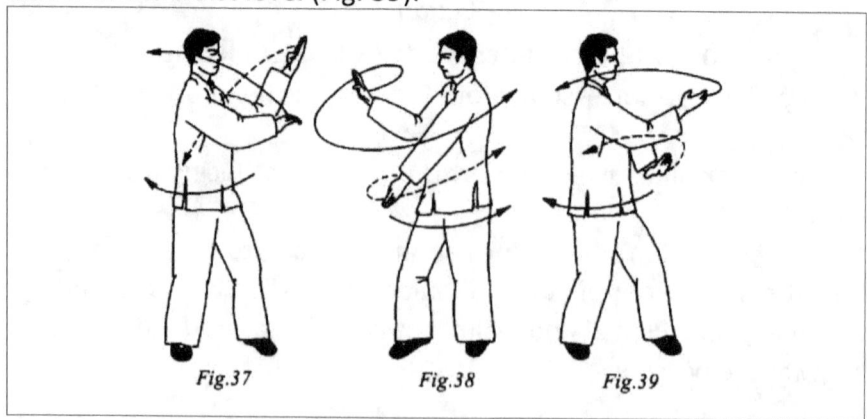

Fig.37   Fig.38   Fig.39

7. Continue to make an inhale. Hands do not change their position. Torso turns to the right. After that, lift your hands up a little (Fig. 40).

8. Turn the right palm to the area of the upper Dantian. Move the hand from the trough adjacent to the outer corner of the left eye, past the left shoulder, chest, left elbow, left lower part of abdomen to the right lower part of abdomen. At the same time, expand the left palm from you and make the movement of the forearm around the elbow on a circle to the left and down, then right and up. Torso turns to the left. The movement is made at the exhale (Fig.41, 42).

9. Turn forward, put hands on the area of the lower Dantian and take the stance of "Growing of the internal pill" (Fig.43).

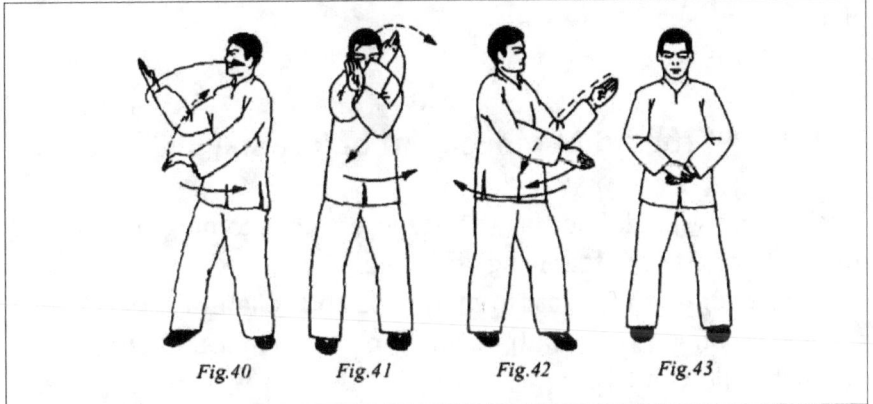

Fig.40   Fig.41   Fig.42   Fig.43

Complete three or nine breaths (exhale - inhale).

Important points:

1. When the hand is turned palm up, you must imagine that you gather "Celestial Qi».

When the hand is turned palm down, you must imagine that you gather "Earth Qi».

Thus you gather "Celestial and Earth Qi".

2. Turn the hand palm to the area of the upper Dantian, you must imagine that the gathered Qi penetrates the point between the eyebrows ("Celestial Eye»-Tianmu) and from there it descends along the "Wonderful meridians".

When you make a circular movement with the other hand, imagine that at this time the "Turbid Qi» removes.

Explanations:

This exercise strengthens the ability to "Spiritual perception", and also allows to collect "Pure Qi" and delete "Turbid Qi". Turning one palm up, and the other - palm down during the actions of moving the hands on the arc has the aim to "Mastering the spiritual Qi of Sky, Earth and Ten thousand things". During the turning the hand palm up to "Celestial Chambers" of the upper Dantian,«Spiritual Qi »penetrates the Tianmu point, which is a kind of door to the subtle world. Circular motion with a hand in front of the body involves the removal of "Turbid Qi». This facilitates the penetration of "Pure Qi" of the human to the brain and lowering "Turbid Qi" down. This increases the human intellectual possibilities and inspired state of mind.

Section 4
"The art of movement of internal pill"

This exercise is defined as the stage of "Overcoming the middle outpost" and has the following objectives:

1. Improvement the cross of meridians and collaterals.

2. Overcoming of "Outposts" - places where there is an obstructed flow of Qi energy.

3. Increase of joint mobility.

"Nine circulations to improve patency of collaterals"
Turns of neck

1. Starting position - "The position of growing of internal pill".

2. Draw your hands down, palms are turned forward. Raise your hands up in an arc along the sides of the torso, place your palms on the back of the neck. Pinkies are on the Fengchi points, located under the back of the head, in the fossa bone behind the ear at the level of the ear canal. The rest of the fingers touch the neck. Palms touch the front surface of the mandible (Fig.44).

3. With a slow motion tilt your head forward and down. Simultaneously make an exhale (Fig.45). After this with a slow motion lift your head to its original position, then overturn it back. At the same time make an inhale.

4. Make the rotation of the head in a circle. The movement begins with the head rotation to the left. Make three or nine full turns in a clockwise direction. The first half of the turnover – is n inhale, the second half of the turnover – is an exhale (Fig.46).

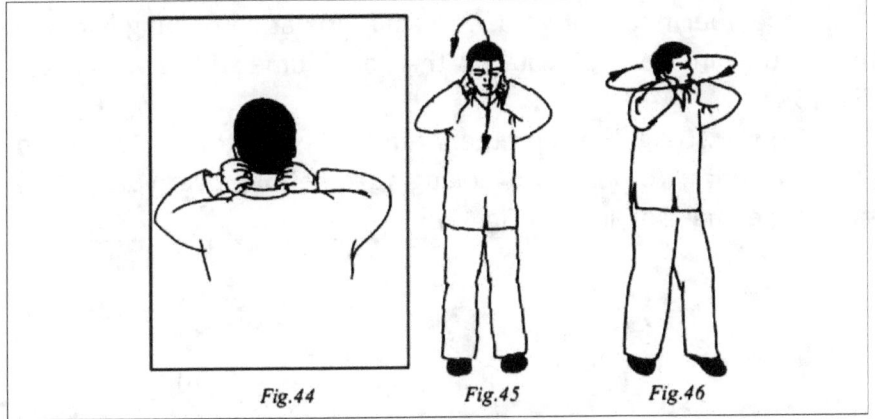

Fig.44   Fig.45   Fig.46

Important points:

1. Upper part of the torso must be stationary.

2. The role of the "axis" in the turns and tilts of the head is neck.

3. Tilts and rotating of the head should be made slowly and with a maximum amplitude.

4. While pressing the acupuncture points do not use physical force, capable to prevent the relaxation or withdrawal from rest state and concentration.

Explanations:

This exercise provides the mobility of the cervical spine area and unlocking the top "Outpost" area. Impact of fingers on the acupuncture points on the neck plays the role of a massage by pressure method. Tilts of the head forward as if "pull" Qi at the back – mid Du-mai meridian, which contributes to its upward movement. Turnover of the head back "covers" the zone of the Da zhui GV-14 point, between the last cervical and first thoracic vertebrae, which contributes to the concentration of Qi in this area. Alternate bending and tilting of the head lead to a greater concentration of Qi energy and overcoming the top "outpost". Qi as if "stretches" and then abruptly "compresses", giving the impetus to move forward in the direction of its flow. Head rotation is associated with "Celestial circle".

Bending of the torso at the waist

1. From the starting position lower your arms down and grasp the waist at the sides. Thumbs are placed on Shenshu UB-23 points (Fig.47).

2. Bend your body forward. You as if look at something lying on the ground in front of you. At the same time, make an exhale (Fig.48).

3. Slowly straighten up, then tilt back the torso. The head overturns back. You are as if looking at something over you. At the same time, make an inhale (Fig.49).

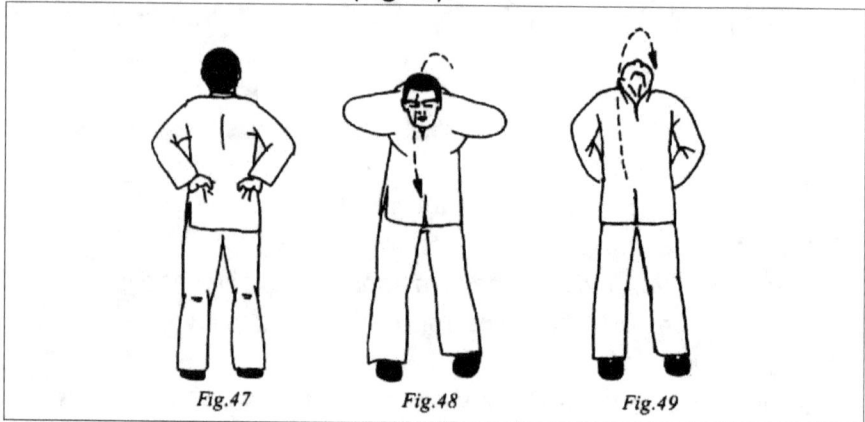

Fig.47   Fig.48   Fig.49

The exercise is made three or nine times.

Important points:

1. *During the bending and deviations you must keep the body straight.*

2. *Center of the movement is back.*

3. *during making the exercises you should avoid the overvoltage of legs at the knee joints.*

Rotation of the body

This exercise is a continuation of the previous exercise.

Using waist as the axis of rotation, bend the body forward, then rotate the torso in the clockwise direction (forward, left, backward, right, forward).

At the first half-turn of the body make an inhale, at the second half of the turnover - exhale.

Do this exercise three or nine times.

"Swinging of the hands"

1. Starting position - "the position of growing of the internal pill" (Fig.50).

2. Availably lower your arms down. The palms turnto the front of the thighs. Make an exhale (Fig.51).

3. At the inhale with a slow motion lift both hands up to the level of average Dantian. Palms are turned to you, fingers are pointing down.

4. Using the waist as the axis of rotation, turn the body to the left. Hands move in an arc down-left-up and rise to the horizontal level in front of the chest in front of the average Dantian. Simultaneously make an exhale (Fig. 52).

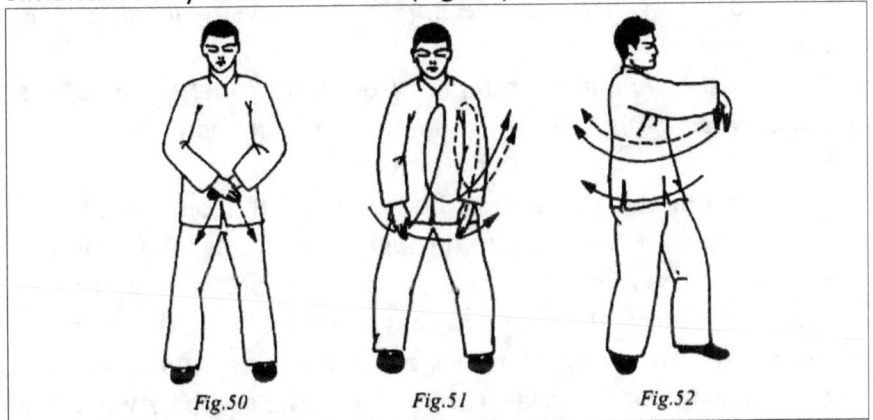

Fig.50   Fig.51   Fig.52

5. Similarly to the previous motion, turn the body to the right. Hands move in an arc to the right-down-up to the horizontal level and are located in the area of the average Dantian. At the same time, make an inhale (Fig.53).

6. Similarly to the previous movement, turn the body to the left. Hands move in an arc to the left – down -up, to the horizontal level and are located opposite the average Dantian. At the same time, make an inhale (Fig.54).

Make the exercise nine times, counting for one cycle "inhale-exhale".

7. Turn the face forward and lower your hands, put the palms on the area of the lower Dantian. You are in the original position "position of growing of the internal pill" (Fig.55).

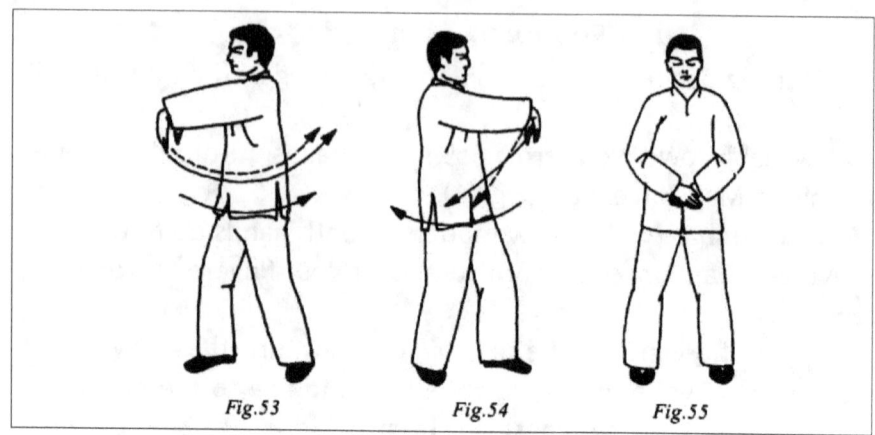

Fig.53   Fig.54   Fig.55

Important points:

1. During the swinging of the hands, the movements should be slow and gradual.

2. During the changing of stances from right to left-handed, the hand movements must be carried out in an arcuate path.

Explanations:

During making the above described exercise, the joint mobility of the lumbar spine increases. The throughput of the Qi energy in the back-middle Du-mai meridian in the Jiajia "outpost" area improves. The torso turns at the waist with a relaxation in the average "outpost" area are a kind of massage of the kidneys and abdominal viscera. Activate the "Mobile Qi" centered in the space between the kidneys and establish the interaction between Dantian and Mingmen areas.

Chapter 4
Static Qigong exercises

After the Dynamic exercises of Qigong are mastered, you should pass to the study of the Static exercises.

The purpose of the Static exercises of Qigong is the melting of the "Inner pill" without movement.

The trainings are divided into six stages:

1. *"Regulation"*
2. *Focusing on the area of the lower Dantian*
3. *Moving Qi from the lower Dantian to the average Dantian*
4. *Gathering of "Three Flowers" on the top, "Melting of the spirit" and "Achieving emptiness"*
5. *The final exercise*
6. *Return to a normal state of consciousness.*

"Regulation"
1. "Regulation of the body"

Sit down, bend your knees and take a half lotus position, lotus or cross-legged. Keep your head straight, the Baihui point should be directed upwards. Eyes are covered. Tongue touches the palate behind the alveoli. Lower the shoulders and elbows, relax the underarm area. Both hands are put on each other in such a way as the Laogong points projected on each other. Men put the right hand at the top women- left. Hands are located on the area of the lower Dantian. Relax your lower back.

Make a deep inhale and with the exhale relax your body from top to bottom. Repeat it three or nine times in a row. Relax your internal organs, focusing first on the head, then on the internal organs, the chest area, abdomen, and bone marrow.

When the muscles, joints and the whole body will be relaxed, you will have a feeling of an unusual lightness.

At the inhale, lift the Qi energy from the Huiyin point to the Baihui point, then make an exhale and at the same time lower the Qi from the Baihui point to the Huiyin point. These two points have to be connected as if with the straight line.

2. Establishing the breathing

During this exercise it is necessary to use the reverse abdominal breathing. You should make nine breathing cycles.

3. Establishing the consciousness

With the help of "Establishing the body" and "Establishing the breathing" you can reach a state of peace. You should be free from extraneous thoughts. The consciousness becomes like the calm water. Body and internal organs relax, Qi and blood are lowered, "Seed Qi" goes back to its house and the "Emptiness" at the top and "Filling" below are achieved. Baihui and Huiyin points mentally connect to a single line. Nine relaxing breathing cycles are a prelude to the meditative exercises.

"Focusing on the area of the lower Dantian" and "The leading Qi through "Celestial circle"

1. At the exhale, lower Qi to the downward "Vermilion field". A the inhale concentrate Qi in the same area.

At the next inhale in the area of the lower Dantian appears a feeling of appearance of "energy ball". Focus on the downward "Vermilion field." When you feel the pulsation and rotation of the "ball", you can proceed to the next exercise.

2. Concentrate on the area of the lower Dantian. Power of focus should be relatively small, as if a superficial one. There is a feeling that to the "Vermilion field" starts to receive a certain amount of "Seed energy".

Breathing is easy, type - reverse abdominal (Fig. 1).

3. When "Seed energy" will fill an area of the lower Dantian, it will begin to move on the front - middle Ren-mai and back-middle Du-mai meridian. At first it is necessary to guide the movement of energy thought these meridians. At the inhale Qi from the downward "Vermilion field" must pass through the Huiyin point, then through the Mingmen, Fengfu points, up to the Baihui point.

On the exhale, Qi moves down from the Baihui point on the front-middle meridian passing through the Tiantu, Dan zhong, Shenque - CV8 points and moves back to the lower "Vermilion field" (Fig. 2).

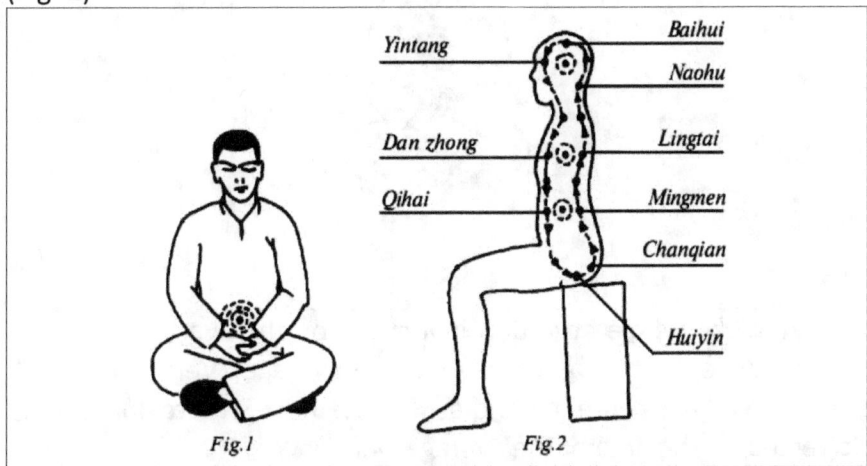

Yintang

Dan zhong

Qihai

Baihui

Naohu

Lingtai

Mingmen

Chanqian

Huiyin

Fig.1   Fig.2

With the growth of skill, energy circulation through the "Celestial circle", happens as if by itself without your mental effort.

Explanations:

Exercises on entering the lower Dantian and the practice of moving of Qi on the "Small celestial circle " – this is a stage in which life ("Seed"), Jing energy is converted into Qi energy. It occurs in three stages: a focus on the downward "Vermilion field" for the concentration of "Seed energy" in it, gathering of "the pill" due to the concentration and mixing of Human Qi, Sky and Earth, saturation of "Vermilion field" "Seed energy" and its spontaneous movement on "Small celestial circle", supported by the idea and breathing. Thus the "Small medicine" is manufactured.

"Moving Qi from the lower Dantian to the average Dantian"

1. At the exhale, lower Qi to the downward "Vermilion field". Thereafter, at the inhale the concentration of attention shifts to the area of average Dantian (solar plexus area), feel that Qi of the whole body is gathering there (Fig. 3).

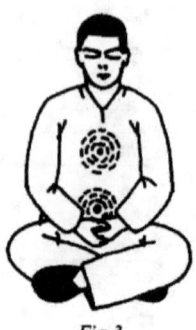

Fig.3

Further, the whole attention is focused on the average Dantian. At the exhale, Qi as if goes beyond the average "Vermilion field" and at the inhale - enters it and as if concentrates there. Inner look is directed on the area of the average Dantian.

You should start with 10-20 minutes of practicing this exercise, and after nine days to bring the exercise time to 30 minutes.

2. Continuing the previous exercise, at the exhale Qi descends to the area of lower Dantian, at the inhale Qi raises again to the average Dantian. Exercise time is 30 - 60 minutes.

Explanations:

At this stage, the melting of Qi energy into the Shen spirit takes place, while the crucible is the lower Dantian. And the average Dantian becomes a tripod. When the technique of moving of vermilion energy from the awerage Dantian to the lower Dantian and vice versa is developed, then the "Golden Pill" will gradually thicken and become the "Big Medicine". At this time, the energy substance might drift along "Great celestial circle" without the help of thought and breathing (Fig. 4 - 10).

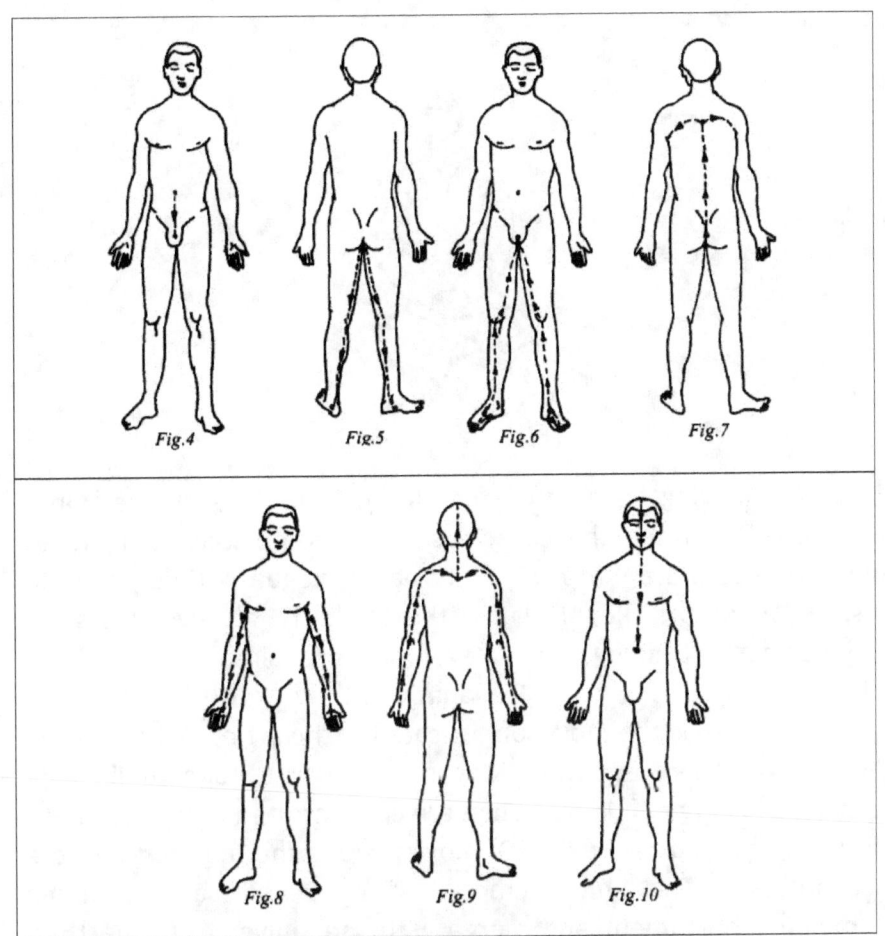

Fig.4   Fig.5   Fig.6   Fig.7

Fig.8   Fig.9   Fig.10

"Gathering three flowers in the top, melting of the spirit and achievement of emptiness"

1. At the inhale lower Qi to the area of lower "Vermilion field". Focus on it. After a few breathing cycles, when "Vermilion field" start to move, at the inhale direct Qi to the upper "Vermilion field."

Focusing is transferred to the Niwangong area, adjacent to the Yintang (Tianmu) point between the eyebrows. Concentration should be very easy, without noticeable efforts (Fig. 11).

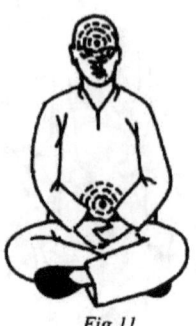

Fig.11

2. After a long training on focusing of attention on the upper Dantian area, when the consciousness is completely calm, takes place a complete stop of "internal dialogue", thoughts and inspiration occurs. People know the truth. To achieve this state quite a lengthy training and perseverance is required.

Explanations:

This exercise is the most sophisticated in the art of melting of the "Inner pill". There are three stages. In the first stage vitality Jing energy, Qi energy and Spirit-Shen are concentrated in the top. With an inner eye you can watch Qi moving along the meridians. In the second stage "The limit of emptiness" is reached - a state of the complete detachment and merge with the Universe. In the third highest stage a complete liberation from thoughts is achieved, intuition manifests and the truth reveals. The understanding of the laws of the Cosmos and human life occurs.

"The final exercise"

Discontinue the exercise on concentration of attention. Mentally say nine times: "I am relaxed."

"Return to normal state after exercises"

1. Make rocking with the body 9 or 36 times in a clockwise direction and the same amount of times in a counterclockwise direction.

2. Make massage of knees, ankles, upper limbs and face.

Chapter 5
Basics of "Energetic" massage

In the Tianzhu shan Qigong system are actively applied the energy massage techniques. After some time of training, the training person gets an opportunity to develop the "External Qi" and using it to affect certain areas of the body. Energetic massage using the "External Qi" is made with the following of requirements: relaxing, immersing of the consciousness in a "state of Qigong", precise localization of effects, ease and fluidity of movements. In the initial stages of the practice, the massage is made by direct contact exposure on areas of the body, in consequence, when the ability to enhance the flow of "External Qi» comes, the impact can be very easy, and at the higher stages of massage is performed with the help of "Promise Qi", without a direct contact with body.

Exercise 1

"The impact on the Yongquan - KD1 point"

In a sitting position with the crossed legs bend the massaged leg at the knee. Put the palm of the right hand with the Laogong - PC8 point on the Yongquan point of the left foot. With rubbing back and forth motions massage the specified area, making eighty one movements (Fig. 1). Similarly, make massage of the other leg.

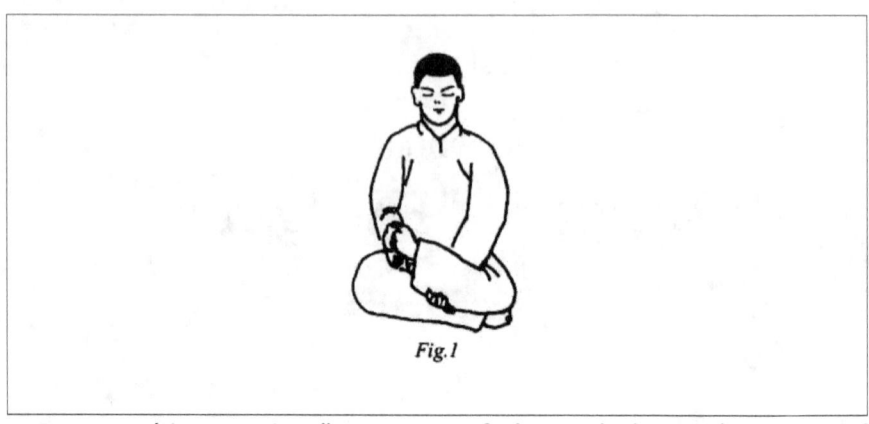

Fig.1

Due to this exercise "Lowering of the turbid Qi», lowering of blood pressure, establishment of the interaction between the heart and kidneys, etc. occur.

Explanations:

The Yongquan - KD1 points relate to the Kidney meridian. Through them, the contact with "Earth Qi» is made, serving as a kind of "Gates" through which energy enters the human organism.

The Laogong - PC8 points relate to the Pericardium meridian. The contact between Laogong and Yongquan points involves joining of heart and kidneys through their related meridians. To the "Fire" of Heart corresponds the Li trigram, and to the "Water" of kidney - Kan trigram. Thus, "Water" and "Fire" relate to each other on the basis of interaction of Kan and Li trigrams.

Exercise 2

"The impact on the kidneys area"

Place the palms with Laogong points on the back on the areas, located at the level of the gap between the spinous processes of the third and fourth lumbar vertebrae, to the side for one and a half Cuns. Make thirty six friction up and down movements (Fig. 2).

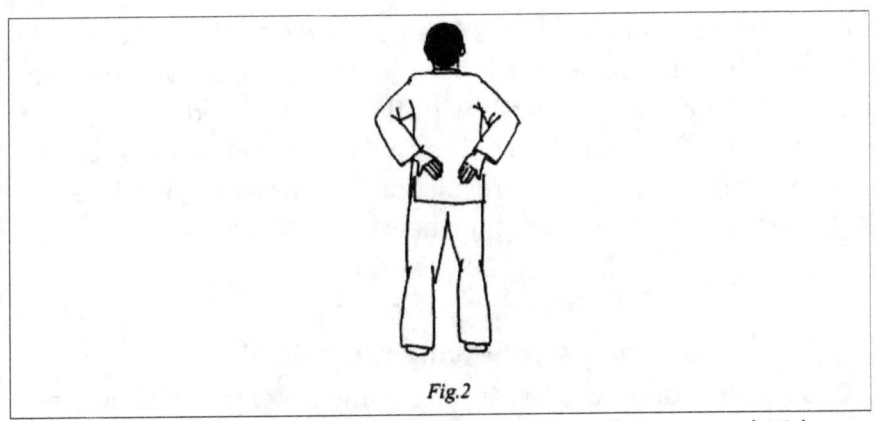

Fig.2

Due to this exercise, there is a connection of Heart and Kidneys, strengthening of the kidneys and lumbar muscles.

Explanations:

The impact occurs in Shenshu points area, relating to the foot Shaoyin meridian. The Laogong points refer to the arm Pericardium meridian. Contact of these points provides the interaction of Heart and Kidneys by the type of relations between the Kan and Li trigrams - «Water support the Fire".

Exercise 3

"Tapping the teeth"

With light rhythmic movements make thirty six taps with the teeth. During this exercise strengthening of teeth, gums and kidneys occur.

From the point of view of the Chinese medicine the kidneys control the state of the skeletal system. Tapping with teeth stimulates Qi of kidney, which in turn helps to strengthen the bones and bone marrow playback.

Exercise 4

"The excitement of the sea"

With your tounge make thirty six rotating, mixing movements. During this exercise the stimulation of salivation, cleansing the mouth, the regulation of heart rate and visceral functions occur.

Explanations:

From the point of view of the Chinese medicine tip of the tongue is associated with the heart and lungs, and its edges - with the liver and gall bladder, central part - with the stomach and spleen, back area - kidney. In accordance with this, the movements of the tongue contribute to the regulation of visceral functions, in particular - "filling of blood" of the heart rate.

Exercise 5

"Washing the mouth
and swallowing the saliva"

Close your mouth and "cleanse" the mouth with saliva. Make it thirty times, then swallow the saliva. During this exercise activation of salivation, oral cleansing and antiseptic of stomach occur.

Explanations:

As saliva has antiseptic properties, during the exercise it performs an anti-inflammatory effect on the gums, teeth, and when swallowing, replenishes the Yin-substance of the body.

Exercise 6

Impact to the forehead

Place the hands with palms on the forehead and make thirty six friction up and down movements (Fig. 3). The effect of this exercise is shown in combating of wrinkles, mental relaxation and getting rid of the pain in the frontal area of the head.

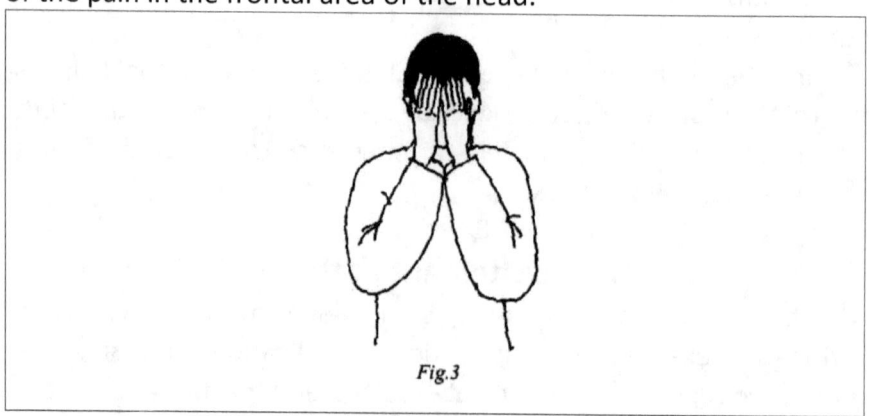

Fig.3

Explanations:

In the Chinese medicine it is believed that the forehead area is classified to Yangmin - «Bright Yang», which is concentrated in the area of the Tianmu point. Massage of the forehead promotes the free circulation of Qi through the Yangmin meridians and resolves the headaches caused by stagnations in Yangmin substances.

Exercise 7

"Dry washing"

Place the palms on the face, and make thirty six friction up and down movements (Fig. 4). The effect of this exercise is to prevent the appearance of wrinkles and strengthen the muscles of the face.

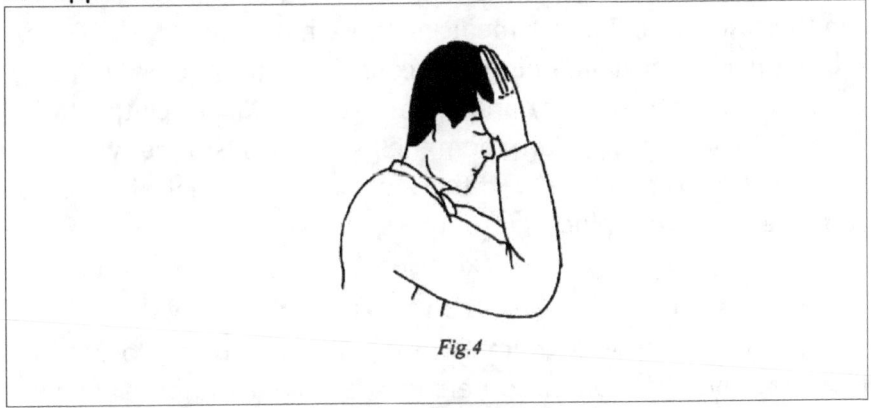

Fig.4

Explanations:

It is believed that through twelve main meridians and three hundred sixty-five of collaterals blood and Qi come to the face and fill all the pores of the skin. As a consequence, a beneficial effect on the internal organs, meridians and collaterals of the whole body occur.

Exercise 8

"The impact on the nose"

Place the fingers of both hands on the face so that the tips of the middle fingers are on the sides of the nose grooves (Yingxiang - Li20 point). Make thirty six rubbing movement with middle fingers from the Yingxiang points to the Yintang point between the eyebrows and back (Fig. 5, 6).

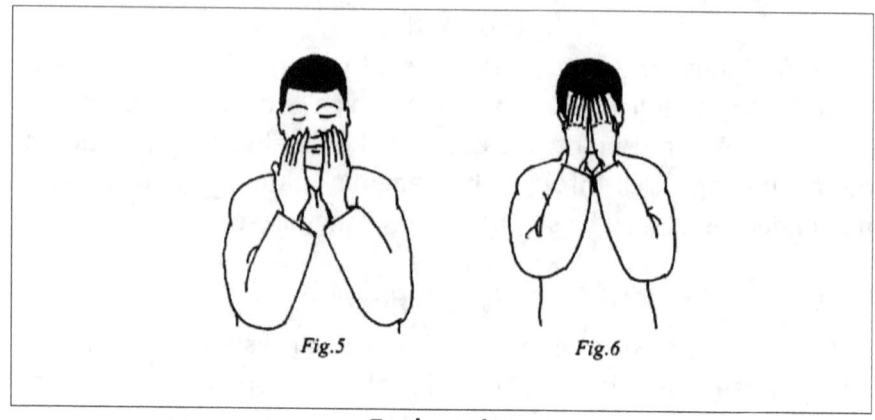

Fig.5　　　　Fig.6

Explanations:

In the traditional Chinese medicine, nose has a name: "The Gates of breathing". Yingxiang points are considered the 'Holes', relating to the wings of the nose, and the Yintang point – "Outpost" of "Celestial eye". Impact on them helps to cleanse the ways of movement of "Lengths Qi" and therefore the treatment of diseases connected with the "blockage" of these routes.

Exercise 9

"The impact on area of Tai Yang points"

Place the tips of your thumbs on the Tai Yang point, located in the valleys near the outer corners of the eyes. Bend other fingers and push to the forehead. With circular motions of the thumbs, massage the area of the Tai Yang points. First, make thirty six movements from the inside-out, then the same amount in the opposite direction (Fig. 7).

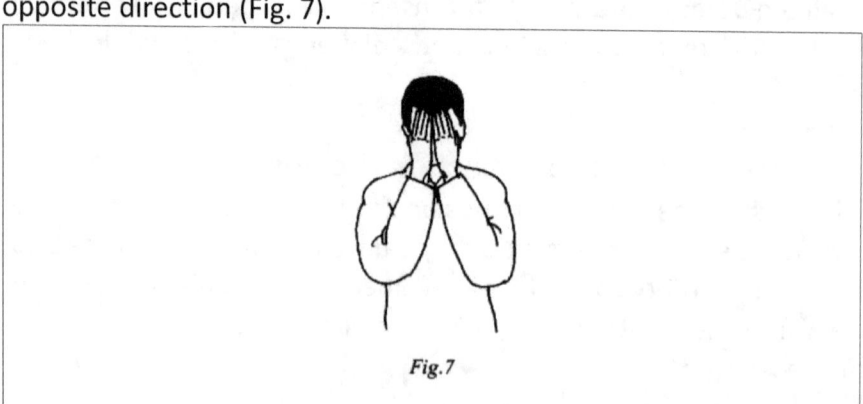

Fig.7

The massage of areas of Tai Yang points relieves mental stress, prevents and cures pain in the temporal area, improves the circulation of blood and Qi in around the eye area.

Exercise 10

"The impact on the earlobes"

Grasp the ears so that your thumbs are behind the ears, with the rest fingers bent in the joints make stroking downward movement thirty-six times (Fig. 8). Then similarly make thirty - six stroking movements in the earlobes area (Fig. 9).

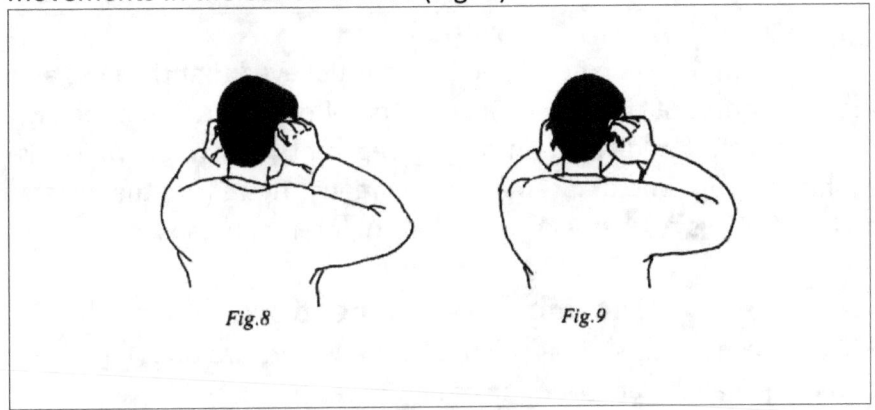

Fig.8   Fig.9

Explanations:

Ear area is connected with the internal organs through the energy meridians. Stroking of curls and earlobes affects the located on them acupuncture points and helps to regulate the functions of internal organs.

Exercise 11

"Impact on the eye area"

Close your eyes. Put the tips of the middle fingers on the eyelids, make thirty - six light circular massaging movements clockwise, then a similar amount of massaging movements in the counterclockwise direction. Then make thirty - six rotational movements of the eyeballs to one, then the other side (Fig. 10, 11).

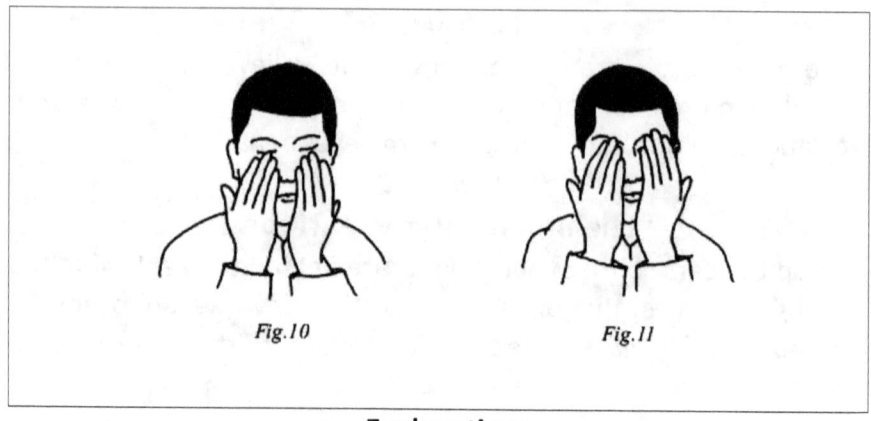

Fig.10   Fig.11

Explanations:

In the traditional Chinese medicine it is believed that the eyes are the focal point of the "Seed Qi" of internal organs. Conventionally, the eye can be divided into five segments, each of which is connected with one of internal dense organs. Therefore, the impact on the eyeballs regulates the functions of internal organs.

Exercise 12

"The impact on the head area"

Place both hands so that the tips of the fingers are on the midline of the head at the anterior line of hair cover (Fig. 12). Tap with your fingertips on the midline of the head removing hands to the back line of hair cover (Fig. 13), then move the hands to the front hairline. Tapping, move the hands along the anterior lineof the hair cover to the pits on the temple, under the hair, at the junction of the frontal and parietal bones (Fig. 14). Next slide down the impact to the temples and to the tips of the ears (Fig. 15) and to the Fengfu point, located back at the bottom of the skull. Repeat the impact route three or nine times.

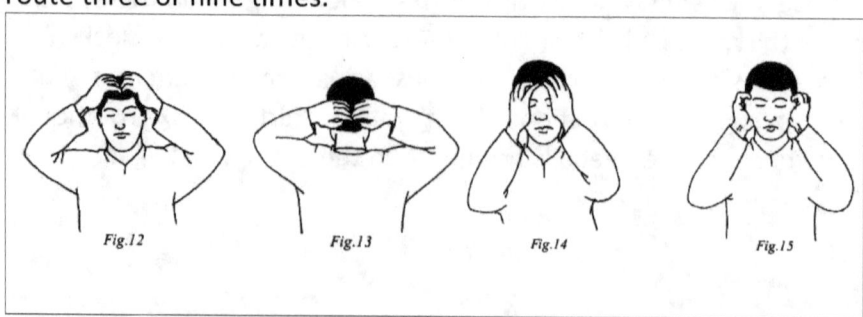

Fig.12   Fig.13   Fig.14   Fig.15

Explanations:

In the traditional Chinese medicine, the head is considered the concentration of Yang substances and "Storage of the brain". As the brain is constantly active, the muscles of the head and are in constant tension, which leads to headaches. Impact on the located on the head acupuncture points makes to relax the head muscles and promotes treatment related to their overexertion of headache. This in turn allows the brain to enter a state of "relaxation".

Tapping with your fingertips on the head improves patency of the backward-middle Du-mai meridian, liberates and activates the upward "Outpost". Accordingly, this exercise promotes the circulation of Qi and blood through the "Celestial circle".

Chapter 6
The general concepts about training

The general concepts present the certain rules and regulations which ensure the maximum effect in the Qigong. They touch the questions of the optimal time for trainings, the clothing, accommodation etc. of the Qigong.

The time of training of the Qigong

The Qigong masters give out four periods a day when the trainings bring the greatest effect: **Qi - shi** (The Hour of the Child) - from 23 o'clock to 1 o'clock p.m., **Wu - shi** (The Noon) - from 11 o'clock to 13 o'clock a. m., **Mao - shi** (The Mao Time) - from 5 to 7 o'clock a. m. and **Yu - shi** (The Yu time) – from 17 to 19 o'clock p. m..

The direction of the training the Qigong

It is believed that the most favorable direction for training of the Qigong is the direction "North – South". You can train the facing to the South, with your back to the North, or opposite, facing to the North, and back - to the South. Since the North is related with the "Water" and the South - with the "Fire", the position of the "facing to the South, back to the North" helps to establish the harmony between them.

Such a position in the relation to the sides of the world is supported in the modern science too. As the person is under the constant influence of the magnetic field of the Earth, the position of the body is oriented towards "North - South", and is coincide with the direction of the lines of force of this field. As the result the magnetism of the human biofield is enhanced, which affects the functioning of the whole organism.

The clothing for training of the Qigong

The clothing should be made of the natural fabric and should not be tightly fitting. If a training person is wearing the clothes made of the synthetic fabric, its excessive electrification prevents the normal flow of the Qi energy. The cloth slippers are preferred. In this case, it is easier to connect with the Earth Qi.

Women should not wear the high heels shoes.

Don't put on the rubber shoes in any case because the rub has insulating properties which prevents the passage of the Qi to the **Yonquan** points.

The Qigong practicing place

You can train indoors in winter and when the weather is cold. In this case, it is important to ensure that the room is ventilated well. The experience shows that if you are training in high-rise apartments (on the 5th floor and above), it will be difficult to contact the Qi of the Earth, so it is recommended to go down.

It is good to train outdoors when it is warm outside.

The greatest effect from the trainings appears during the trainings on forest clearings. This is due to the fact that the trees are living organisms, which for many years has been at the intersection of the relations between the Sky and the Earth. They connect the top and bottom, lead Yin and Yang to the harmony and peace, and have a strong ability to "Collect" and "Splash". Training in the surroundings of the trees, a man gets a good Qi, allocated by them and gives them his sick and throw Qi, which the trees accept.

Nice trees are considered: pine, cypress, poplar, willow, etc. Bad trees are considered the trees near which it is not recommended to train the Qigong: walnut hazel, chestnut, date palm, etc.

The music during the training of the Qigong

During the static trainings of Qigongisit is not recommended to turn on the music, because it would be distracting and counteract the entrance into the standstill.

The restrictions for women

Women should not be engage in Qigong during the menstruation and the pregnancy.

Appendix
The Body Points

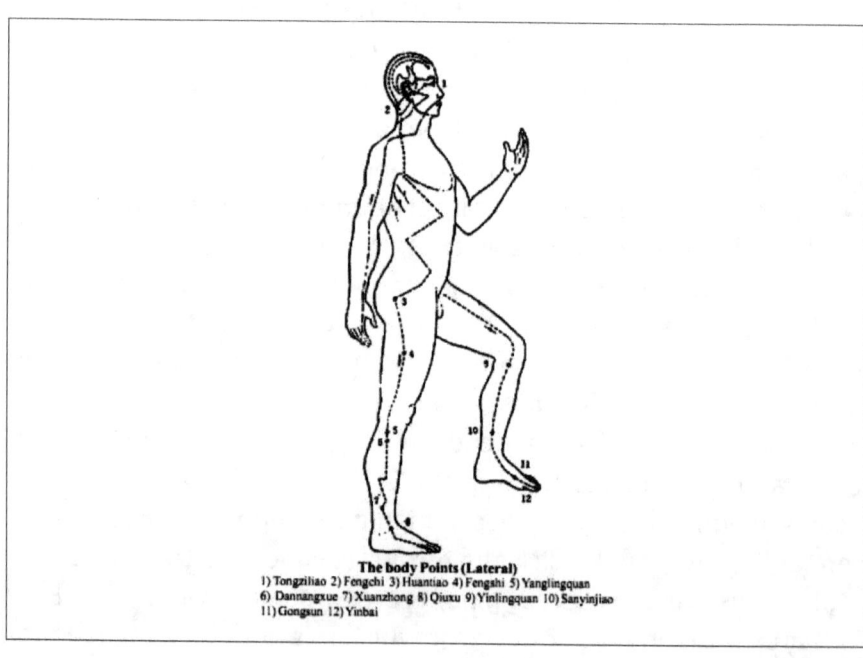

The body Points (Lateral)
1) Tongziliao 2) Fengchi 3) Huantiao 4) Fengshi 5) Yanglingquan
6) Dannangxue 7) Xuanzhong 8) Qiuxu 9) Yinlingquan 10) Sanyinjiao
11) Gongsun 12) Yinbai

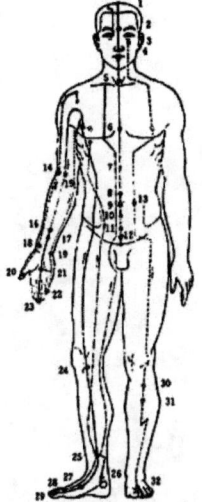

The body Points (Anterior)

1)Baihui 2)Yintang 3) Sibai 4) Suliao 5)Tiantu 6)Shanzhong 7)Zhongwan 8) Shuifen 9) Shenque 10) Qihai 11) Guanyuan 12)Zhongji 13)Tianshu 14) Chize 15)Quze 16) Jianshi 17)Neiguan 18) Lieque 19) Shenmen 20) Shaoshan 21) Laogong 22) Shaochong 23) Zhong chong 24) Yin Lingquan 25) Sanyinjiao 26) Taixi 27) Gongsun 28) Xingjian 29) Yin bai 30)Zusanli 31) Lanwei 32) Neitin

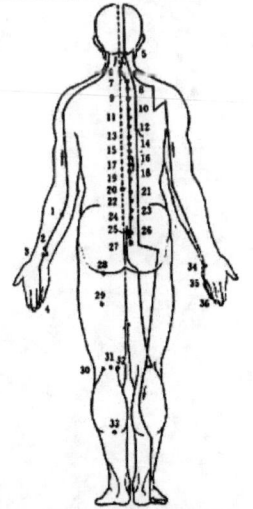

The body Points (Posterior)

1) Sidu 2)Zhigou 3)Waiguan 4) Guanchong 5)Tiantu 6) Dazhui 7)Dashu 8) Fengmen 9) Feishu 10) Jueyinshu 11) Xinshu 12) Dushu 13)Geshu 14) Yishu 15) Ganshu 16) Danshu 17) Pishu 18) Weishu 19) Sanjiaoshu 20) Mingmen 21)Shenshu 22) Qihaishu 23)Dachangshu 24) Guanyuan 25) Ciliao 26) Pangguangshu 27) Baihuanshu 28) Chengfu 29) Yinmen 30) Weiyang 31) Weizhong 32) Yingu 33) Chengshan 34) hand - Wangu 35) Houxi 36) Shaoze

www.ingramcontent.com/pod-product-compliance
Lightning Source LLC
Chambersburg PA
CBHW062019280526
45787CB00005B/2165